LIVE NOW – D.

STARKHEALTH

A dying young doctor travels the world in search of the keys to longevity, health and happiness. Thirty years later – in vibrant health – he has a "Stark" message of hope for all.

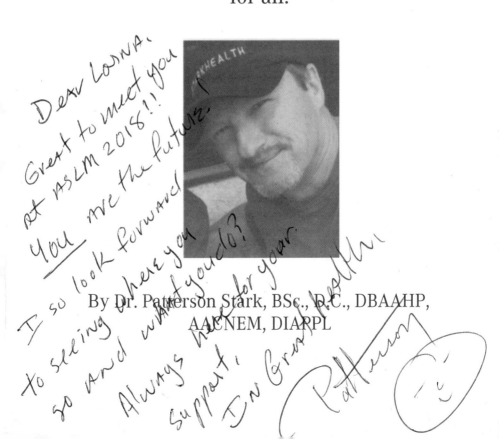

By Dr. Patterson Stark, BSc., D.C., DBAAHP, AACNEM, DIARPL

LIVE NOW – DIE LATER
STARKHEALTH

Published by STARK-MEDIA, a division of StarkHealth Ltd.
4/23 Humphreys Drive, Christchurch, New Zealand
www.StarkHealth.com
+64 03 376 5000
First printing China, October 2010
Second Edition, 2015,

ISBN 978-0-473-16408-9

Dedication

This book is dedicated to the lasting memory of Dr. Paul White, D.C., DICAK of Douglas, Wyoming, who passed away in October 2009. He was a great mentor, friend, educator, businessman, author, rancher, father, grandfather, and loving husband to his wife Marcia. He is a large part of my story, never wavering in support for the 33 years since we met. He will be missed deeply and never to be replaced in the fields of Chiropractic and Therapeutic Nutrition. He was distinguished amongst his neighbors and peers.

Contents

Foreword

By Stephen T. Sinatra, MD, FACC

Patterson Stark's book *Live Now Die Later* is a must-read for anyone with a health challenge – especially cancer, heart disease, and the wrath of other "chronic" illnesses of our modern lifestyle. It's equally essential to anyone who loves or lives with a person diagnosed with any of these conditions, as well as any professional caring for them. Actually, it's even a basic primer for any of us looking to prevent illness from happening in the first place. We all need this book!

Dr Stark's message is clear, concise, and to the point, and his perspective is pretty unique. You see, Dr. Stark is a medically trained professional who was diagnosed with testicular cancer himself over twenty-nine years ago, while only a young man in his thirties. He followed the guidelines of traditional cancer therapy to the letter: surgical excision of the site of the cancer and "chemo". Chemotherapy has a very high success rate for his particular kind of cancer.

Despite his best efforts, Stark came to realize that he needed to change tactics quickly lest he be forced to confront the "Grim Reaper." His cancer was not responsive to treatment; it had gotten the upper hand. At first he panicked, as would anyone. Knowing the only recourse was to take matters into his own hands after failed chemotherapy, Stark was forced to think "outside the box" if he was to survive. Eventually, he was able to put a positive spin on the situation at hand, and view it as an "opportunity in crisis." Dealing with the possibility of an untimely death, Stark would come around to feel the essence of what it really is to be "alive."

To "beat cancer", or any other disease, you must take back control of your own life. Success means following some specific basic strategies: a healthy lifestyle; detoxifying the body; maintaining a non-inflammatory, non-insulin provoking diet; taking targeted nutritional supplements; and seeking the advice of others that you trust. In my experience, the "Super Perfecta" for cancer survival, in simplest of terms, is this: no sugar, plenty of oxygen, detoxification, and a positive intention.

In order to survive cancer, you must also explore the multifaceted aspects of your emotional, physical, and spiritual feelings. Dr. Stark's tactics also engaged the healing aspects that nature has to offer. He recognized the value of maintaining positive intentions and reinforcing a belief in the self. He reaffirmed his faith in the body's innate wisdom to know how to heal itself when given the appropriate support.

Stark's recovery and cure serve as an inspiration to anyone with cancer or anyone dealing with any catastrophic illness, for that matter. In my professional opinion, he did it right. If others employ the same "StarkHealth" approach to recovery and wellness, most catastrophic illnesses can be avoided – in fact, Dr. Stark's ongoing research confirms this clinically. This is the Stark message and the Stark solution!

As a clinical cardiologist who's attended the bedside of hundreds of critically ill people, I have oftentimes listened to their reflections. I learned from them that major catastrophic illnesses most often are placed in one's path for a reason. As life is thrown into a kind of "suspended animation" mode, people are often forced to slow down from their busy lives and pause to evaluate their life choices...

Sometimes it takes a catastrophic illness to literally open us up to discover a new understanding of life. And at other times, we may fall prey or victim to an illness that ends in the death of our physical being.

But why is the treatment of chronic illness – cancer included, so difficult for so many of us? And why haven't we progressed over the last four decades? Cancer, as an example, continues to pervade, control, and destroy lives now as much as it did 40 years ago. The long-term survival rates for people with advanced lung, colon, rectal, breast, and prostate cancer have hardly budged since the war on this deadly disease was declared in 1971. Whereas 100 years ago only 1 in 30 people would develop cancer, nowadays the incidence is 1 in 3 people.

The way things are headed, it won't be long before we'll see cancer surpass heart disease to become the leading cause of death in the United States. Eventually, cancer will literally kill every other person in this country, unless we change our detection and treatment approaches.

In spite of billions of dollars spent on clinical research into the effectiveness of pharmaceutical agents, progress and survival continue to be thwarted. Many recent leading-edge drugs may possibly extend one's lifespan by several weeks or months, but the cost is huge.

Many conventional therapies often have devastating side effects that can be life-debilitating as well as life-threatening. Although over the last couple of decades there has been significant progress in the conventional treatment of some cancers – particularly childhood leukemia, as well as some lymphomas and testicular cancer – chemotherapy has not really proven to be as efficacious as we had hoped for most cancers. The relentless utilization of chemotherapeutic agents by the pharmaceutical industry and physician promotion of the chemotherapy arsenal have both perpetuated the myth that drugs are the end-all-be-all cure for cancer.

The exaggerated marketing in the media perpetuates an expectation and a hype that far outstretches the actual benefits of traditional cancer treatments. Many drug manufacturers cannot prove that their agents prolong survival. They continue to emphasize changes in lab measurements as proof that they work – such as reduction in tumor size or variations in biochemical blood markers. Actually, fluctuation of tumor size is not evidence of a drug's efficacy, and sadly doesn't always correlate with cure, let alone any benefit to quality of life.

Although most conventional cancer treatments are founded upon a "cut, burn, and poison" philosophy, surgery, radiation, and chemotherapy collectively have serious limitations. Surgical procedures that remove localized structured tumors that have not metastasized can indeed save lives. But radiation and chemotherapy therapies must be considered suspect. The methods we use to diagnose as well as evaluate conventional chemotherapy treatments must also be questioned.

Most folks don't realize that a person receiving a typical CT scan of the abdomen, for example, will receive about the same radiation as a Hiroshima survivor of World War II. The radiation exposure incurred during routine mammography may also increase a woman's risk for developing breast cancer, especially if she continues to have serial mammograms.

Researchers have cautioned us that when people are treated with chemotherapy and radiation, it could also increase their risk of a subsequent or new cancer by 20-fold. Cancer centers don't routinely pass along that warning. Thus, finding safer diagnostic as well as therapeutic modalities should be a high priority in this country; but is it? Natural remedies and alternative therapies are potent resources for prevention and treatment. But how often are they considered by the present medical establishment?

The answer to those questions is sadly simple: not so often. Why? Politics and economics...

Since naturally occurring substances like vitamins, herbs, enzymes, and so forth cannot be patented, there's no real money to be made by Big Pharma or big business. Pharmaceutical companies won't be investing in the R&D for these natural therapies any time soon because it is not in their best interest economically. Why challenge drugs that are already earning billions of dollars? Clearly the rules of economics dominate the trend in cancer that we have been seeing for the last 40 years.

And politically speaking, there are more well-paid lobbyists for the pharmaceutical industry worldwide than any other single interest, so disturbing the status quo of this private interest group is nothing I expect to see in my lifetime. The push for alternative solutions must come from the people themselves... with leaders like Patterson Stark.

I truly believe that most physicians work in the best interest of patient welfare. Most of these same physicians truly believe that their treatment works despite failure after failure; how else would they be able to sleep at night? Unfortunately, they unknowingly collude with the myth that conventional pharmaceutical treatments are the only therapy of choice. It's all they have to offer. Deep down, though, many cancer docs long for more comprehensive and promising solutions. I know; they talk to me about their hopes and dreams to save more patients.

But there is hope, as Stark points out in *Live Now - Die Later, Starkhealth*. He has experienced firsthand that conventional and alternative therapies can converge to make a real difference in cancer survival. After all, Stark is living proof of his methods. He is a "sixty-something" Chiropractic Physician with 9% body fat, an impressive mental acumen and he walks the walk! This book should be read by anyone who is developing a chronic illness battle plan. Ultimately, Stark asks us to search for meaning not only in survival, but also in life itself – so that we can walk the walk of health in our own unique individual way.

Stark invokes ancient sciences that are as valid as quantum physics "in my fight to stay on the planet." He talks of compassion as a realization of one's actions having significant impacts on the well-being of others. Patterson Stark stares cancer right in the eye and looks at it from the cellular level, which is similar to the way I treat heart disease. I rely on metabolic interventions that support energy substrates in the cell, an approach that I refer to as "metabolic cardiology." Stark has evoked the theories of Otto Warburg for healing. It's Warburg's theory that cancer thrives on sugar and languishes in an oxygen rich environment. Simple bottom line if we "humanize" the cancer cell: cancer loves sugar and hates oxygen. Stark really resonated with that insight.

By dismissing sugars from his diet, and increasing oxygenation with exercise, Stark's solution dismantled the key agent that feeds cancer, and supported an environment that starves it at the same time.

Cancer cells can metabolize up to 19 times more glucose than healthy cells, and they keep busy dividing and conquering in a low oxygen (anaerobic) environment. So, it's a no-brainer that when anyone with cancer cuts off its food supply – sugar – the cancer will suffer. When simultaneously, oxygen levels are ramped up in the body through aerobic activities like exercise, hyperbaric oxygen (HBOT), and/ or targeted nutraceutical support (like IV vitamin C which supports oxygenation), it's a one-two punch. Keep up that plan, and eventually you've got your knockout punch!

Clearly, when one is in an active cancer battle, processed and/or sugary foods, as well as high-glycemic fruits and alcohol, must be completely avoided. Meat products that have been radiated, insecticides, pesticides, and other industrial chemicals must be avoided as well. What is there left to eat? Plenty! Plate up on wild migratory salmon or free-range meats such as chicken and bison for healthy protein sources. An 80 percent organic, plant-based diet is my best recommendation for battling cancer, or even heart disease. It's also the overall best diet to follow for prevention and recovery.

And let us not forget about detoxification. Stark looked at his radiation history from both his father's side and his mother's side. He uncovered many perils that had put him at risk to developing cancer at an early age. It's an eye opener for all of us to consider.

This book will help you identify and neutralize genetic risk factors you may carry that can render you more vulnerable to cancer. Not everyone can be as bold as Stark, who packed up his US-based life and moved to New Zealand, the personal Mecca he selected to increase his chances for survival. But you will learn in this book how to follow his model to set up a healing environment for yourself. Who else does that?

Stark's simple commitment to trust that "love works" is perhaps the strongest fiber in the invisible fabric he weaves to find a higher purpose in life. Stark truly believes, as I do, that positive intention and a belief in yourself and your own healing capabilities will overcome cancer. In my opinion, that's more than one-half the battle.

When you embrace your own healing power, you are on the path to getting well. As a physician for almost 40 years, I have learned to have faith in the "inner physician" in each person. Trust that the body has a profound knowing or "innate intelligence," and when you feed it the metabolic nutrients it needs – healthy, organic food, energized metal-free waters, and targeted nutraceutical supports

– real healing can take place... especially when you have the belief that you will get well!

There is enormous confusion for any patient challenged with a serious illness when given treatment options. Being diagnosed initiates a confusing cascade of choices. Every patient, although advised on many levels, must make their own decisions. Sometimes we need to meditate or pray over what path to take.

I encourage people to educate themselves, study the published research, and build a personal "Stark-healing team." Select family and friends who are loving, supportive, and energizing. Just being around their "chi" will be healing. You may have to suspend your relationships with people that drain your energy – and c'mon, you know who they are – while you heal. Take a break from them until you are well. Pair with doctors and other "healers" who can inform and guide you, and support your individual decisions, even when they may be in conflict with mainstream medical practices.

People with cancer can and should challenge long-standing medical beliefs and personally investigate alternative protocols that can increase their chances of knocking out cancer, as well as manage side effects of chemotherapy and radiation. If you don't know where to begin, find a naturopathic doctor (ND) to add to your team. They can get you started with adjunctive therapies, and educate you about treatment options. Most certified dieticians could guide you if changing the way you grocery shop and eat is a challenge. Cancer Treatment Centers of America, located in several states, have both MDs and NDs on staff.

Sometimes a commitment to a new way of living that enhances emotional and spiritual domains is warranted. Again, I must emphasize that nurturing our core strength and having a strong belief in the potential to cure one's self are as critical to healing as any medicinal treatment whether it be conventional or alternative.

Positive intentions, affirmations, prayer and meditation can help to support our healing energies and empower us. It may be as simple as walking barefoot on the grass.

Patterson Stark's personal battle with cancer is a gut-wrenching struggle with a happy ending. If he can do it, so can you. His insights to mind, body, and spirit are truly noteworthy. In his battle and struggle with cancer, he has lived the rollercoaster ride of agony and ecstasy. His story will touch the heart and soul of all who peruse these pages...

I say follow the StarkHealth message... Live Now and Die Later.

Stephen T. Sinatra, MD, FACC
Brownsville, VT
Author: The Sinatra Solution: Metabolic Cardiology,
Earthing, and co-author, The Great Cholesterol Myth

Preface

From Death's Door to the Wealth of Health

What I did you can do ... benefit from my experience and side-step deadly mistakes!

People feel uncertain about their health. In fact, fear of the unknown has created a society that's in denial about their health, both their present health and their future health.

The Health System is in Chaos

When looking at the causes and odds of how we die, you take a sober look at your own mortality. By doing this, your suspicions will be confirmed: your environment, the system of healthcare you subscribe to, and the strategies you take to avoid disease are all in chaos. Seemingly healthy people are being struck down in the prime of their lives with heart disease, cancer, and the rest of the "headless horsemen of modern disease." The tightening in the pit of your stomach as you read the truth of these words confirms the "Stark-reality."

As a doctor and expert in holistic health, I too was not immune to the lottery of disease. At the age of 34, I was given a diagnosis and it was silently acknowledged that I could have as little as two weeks to live!

Life Becomes Just as Chaotic as the Health System

I vowed that if I did live, I would find the causes of health and happiness. That was a Tuesday. On Thursday, I got the flu. As the death rattle in my body began, so did this story. On Friday, I started chemotherapy. Thirteen weeks later surgical options had to be considered; chemo was not working.

Betting my life, I traveled the planet and found where the keys to longevity, quality of life, and strength were hidden. With all of my resources and limited time, my quest was immediate. I was on a mission to have certainty in my health and live a long life free of dreaded diseases. I wanted to feel vitality, be energetic, and happy with the understanding of how health not only worked but also the assurance that I could be well forever. I wanted to influence the odds in the lottery of life in my favor – if I lived!

How I Can Help You in Your Quest

My own stark resurrection started in 1987. The benefit of this inspirational story is not only to give you hope; you may also find peace of mind. The practices, science, the personal and professional testing on my own body, have taken over 20 years to perfect. By sharing it with you, I can give you a gift of health from the bottom of my heart.

What I learned academically and from experience had to be put into practice in the laboratory of my own life. My patients often report what appears to be a miraculous turnaround in their health and vitality, just from following my Stark Health System and Program for Life. The science supporting it has been hidden from you, the public, and held deep in the books of reason and research. I am living proof of the value of these methods and can expose the real health facts. By doing this, the light of life can enter into your life and with the changes you make, you and also your family will benefit. It's what I call Stark-Simple. I want to take you on a similar journey of discovery of life-changing and health-changing information.

With Humility, Faith and Patience, the Benefits are Great

The study of longevity is thousands of years old. Once I found out that my days were numbered, I went to the ancient ones, asking for direction. I went, humbled. Everything I learned began and ended with faith.

I now challenge you to live a life with certainty about your health by applying these Stark Lifestyle actions.

I can show you how to

- greatly reduce or eliminate your risk of illness

- double your body strength as you effectively train for your age and gender

- leverage your doctors carefully and skillfully, as they, too, are a very real risk factor. (Doctors are the fourth leading cause of death in the United States.)

- choose happiness more often. If you have a sharp and sometimes bitter assessment of the world, it will fade away as a nightmare vanishes.

Life can become easier if you're in a similar predicament. Life is precious and every day is a gift. Today I feel that it's a gift for me to even offer you this information that came about from my pain and suffering. If you are depressed about your health situation, there are answers. Many of them are the same answers for several health problems. I know that sounds odd, but just read on and you will find them.

Acknowledgements

I acknowledge the great support and wonderful sensitivity that has led me to this place of understanding. The thousands of people that have touched my life in this journey have all played roles in my theater. The play continues and the acts are unending.

My immediate family members were very instrumental in helping. Gayel, who is a monument of compassion and unending support and gave worldly and insightful comment at every stage making it feel like support, not criticism. The other essential and important actors include Mary, my sister; Ray my quiet brother; Tom, my brother-in-law; Marsha, my first love who has added valuable perspective to the first reading as did Brian her partner; Thomas, my nephew and his wife Jessica who teach sensitivity and hope just by being the parents of Francisco my grand-nephew.

Dr. George Goodheart, DC invented Applied Kinesiology, I am forever indebted. Dr. Steve Kaufman, old soul and brother, is one of my oldest friends and most admired minds. He never gives up expanding on the truth of health and what can be done naturally. It is part of his spiritual mission to "put it all together for us." Thank you, Bro.

I acknowledge Bill, my Oncologist, and Dr. Dave Simon (now departed) who seems to show up at pivotal times in my life. Sally Anderson was influential with directness and focus. She is a person to admire and watch as her message of confronting your demons and moving forward helps so many people "detrigger – Free Fall " and get some traction in life and health. Additionally her introduction to Matt Church has sparked a fire. Stuart Rose, my mate who as a wordsmith never stopped asking for quality in my best efforts and is always more than generous with his time for me. Larry Tain,

DC was at ground zero when I was diagnosed with cancer, never giving up support.

Paul and Marcia White have always been there to back any lecture I wanted to give and never stopped giving support; when I was sick they sent life, when I was incomplete, they asked for more. Professional mentors in New Zealand are many and Jacqui Lee Houghton, ND has been a close friend and agile mind to bounce things off of. Of course, Dr. Stephen and Corrine Reiderer, DC, made New Zealand possible with selfless compassion.

Uncle Albert and Aunt Sandy for coming to my graduation, it meant more than you know in 1979 and who now show how good and active you can be in your eight and seventh decades respectively.

My patients who have believed in the message that lifestyle and hard work are the best drugs you can buy and have proven by their work that "Stark Health" is simple, effective, and in some cases lifesaving. My personal assistants made all things possible.

I wish to thank my Lama now departed, Khensur Thabkhey Rempoche whom sits on my right shoulder, his Idem directly responsible for the work started and yet unfinished in this life. Graeme, the lay monk that initiated me to the Tibetan Buddhist teachings of the "Four Noble Truths" must be acknowledged, as should the little man in the bookstore in Sri Lanka who handed me the book, *The Foundations of Mindfulness* many years ago. BV Tridandi Swami, new to my life, has given fresh perspective and delicate clear advice. Hare Krishna my friend. My parents are now gone as well as my stepfather; all have played in the richness of this life. All are blessings; however, none of these are as big as my blessings of tumors and scars that have awakened in me the desire to change, to adapt and move on emotionally, physically, and spiritually. "From great intention comes great results!" said John Klemmer and I believe it – no, I demand it!

Dr. Stephen T. Sinatra, MD, FACC has traveled the road of truth and listened with compassion to his patients as they asked for help. This led him to the field of Nutrition and Psychology. Bravely, he has posed uncomfortable questions to his colleagues and fought hard against apathy, ignorance, and condemnation. The first time I heard his words, I understood this. In fact, I went up to him and told him I had appreciated the battle and also had fought in the same war on ignorance. He heard me out of the crowd and over the next couple of years I was drawn deeper into the depth of Dr. Sinatra's knowledge. My most sincere feelings of gratitude go to Dr. Sinatra, his wife Jan and their remarkable son, Stephen. The world is a much better place with them in it.

Everything is related; this is a Stark-reality repeated in my life. You will find it true in your life also.

Dr. Donna Schwontkowski has edited this book, without her it would still be an idea lost in space. She was so patient with me and "coached" this project to a higher level.

Jeff Rudolph, who did an outstanding job on the proof reading the second edition and cleaning up my syntax from living on multiple continents. I look forward to your bight future!

Special thanks to Garik Barseghyan for the cover layout, Lisa Thomson and Sharon Royal, my secretaries, for proofing the final manuscripts over and over, and Heidi Anderson for the back cover photo.

Sarva mangalum, (All blessings),
Patterson
Christchurch, New Zealand, April, 2010, 2015

Introduction

Life can be funny. There are lessons to learn along the way that take each one of us in directions never really dreamed of before. I think of each day as an education, but I have also amassed a comprehensive education in multiple fields of medicine, anthropology, public health, chiropractic, Chinese medicine, Ayurvedic medicine, psychology, martial arts, architecture, farming, animal husbandry, furniture making, paragliding, Buddhism, and Taoism. All my educational pursuits were self-centered in an effort to save my life with the hope of finding a sense of certainty and happiness.

I turn from self-centeredness now to reaching out to you with this knowledge. Hoping you understand how *important* this is to you, your quality of life, and the possibility of health certainty.

I traveled the world, observed and participated in all that would benefit my goal to live another six months. What was planned and what actually occurred is the story of my life – so far. It is rich with irony, satire, humility, and humor. Truth has a way of being painful or beautiful, depending on how you look at it.

My pain can now become your benefit. Even if my life story may be vastly different than your life, we both have something in common: our human physiology. Things that affect me physically and lead to disease will also do the same to you, because you are human. It's this common thread that motivates me so deeply to reach out.

My story is a collection of small stories that make up my life, death, and my life now as I teach. If you need to hop around in the book or are in a situation that you feel is making you panic about your health, start with getting all white processed food out of your diet. In no more than the time it would take to view a long movie, you will have made it through the whole book and have a proper perspective. Ponder the lessons I learned and they will help you change your health and your life too.

But there is a warning that I have for you. Don't ponder the lessons too long. Every day matters, the cycle of self-destruction we have all suffered from continues. Serious poor diet and lifestyle decisions have left many of us with little time. The "Baby Boomers" may just find themselves as the "Exploders" as degeneration accelerates in our later years and becomes rampant. Find the value in these lessons – make it a Stark Awakening – and make changes right now.

There is a real urgency to this message.

With StarkHealth can you *Live Now and Die Later!*

LIVE NOW – DIE LATER

PART ONE

1. *The Moral Imperative – How life beats the truth out of you!*

2. *Colorado Country – Where It All Started*

3. *California – Where It All Ended*

4. *New Zealand – You'll Be Right, Mate!*

5. *Humility – The Raft in the River of Life*

6. *The Ocean of Compassion and the Agony of Ecstasy*

7. *Gratitude – a Reason to Live Better, Longer, and Stronger*

My Story

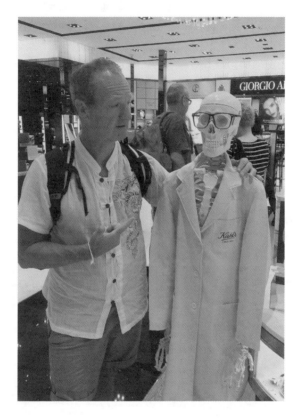

Lest we get too serious remember – it's all a matter
of perspective! Sometimes you just have to laugh;
for that is very good medicine also.

CHAPTER ONE
The Moral Imperative – How life beats the truth out of you!

"Things change, let go of what doesn't work and keep
what does. Have faith. Knowledge exists to help.
Life! Bless it and love the process; it never stops!"
Patterson Stark, D.C.

As corny as it sounds, it all began long, long ago in a universe far, far away...

It was in the fifth year of University that I made the decision to become an architect. Multiple interests from biology to design had filled my years and Humboldt State University had been home for the last three. As I applied to graduate school, I recalled the positive feelings felt during the building of a project and seeing it through to completion. These memories made me realize that it was a fulfilling way of life. Buildings were a perfect metaphor for life and soon, I would be off to Cal Poly State University, San Luis Obispo, California.

Included in my letter of acceptance from the Graduate Department was the standard line, "We are happy to inform you..." and then the tiresome bit about "bringing your mathematics requirements in line with the program." There was also a clause about an "additional year of physics, calculus, and engineering math, which was being added to the Masters program."

My time on campus would now be a three solid year program before I received my Masters... Hmmm. Math was not easy – it was just hard work. I could do it, but it was going to hurt! I went to bed that night thinking only of that backbreaking mathematics in the future.

People will do more to avoid
pain than they will to seek pleasure.

Ask Yourself a Question and an Answer Will Appear

The very next day a phone call came from an old high school water polo buddy. He told me about chiropractic as an alternative to Graduate School. "Chiro-what?" I replied. Sal Arria explained that chiropractic medicine was worth looking into. The previous five years I had worked my way through undergraduate school as a paramedic. It was a means of paying my way and also gave me a closer look at the field of medicine.

Why Enter the Limited Medical Profession?

At first glance, in year one of my University training, I was enamored with the mystique about being "a doctor." However, within a couple of years I concluded that being a medical doctor was not for me. From my vantage point in the emergency room as an emergency medical technician, the medicine I saw was not very creative and was regimented. Politics were evident; creating unnecessary stress within the hospitals and ambulance companies I worked for. I did like the excitement of trauma medicine though, also the creativity of working with my hands and one-on-one with patients. Maybe this chiropractic field really had something to offer?

From what I knew then, chiropractic seemed to be primarily about orthopedics and I liked that. I felt I was good at handling injuries to bones and joints in the field, but what did these guys actually do?

Always Test the Water First

In the next month, I visited a dozen chiropractors. A couple of them were dubious – I couldn't grasp what they actually did. The majority of them however, seemed to be "real doctors." They did not prescribe drugs or do surgery. They did hands-on work and the patients seemed happy. I had no idea this profession even existed; it sounded and looked better all the time.

Decision Making Was Easy

I applied to Los Angeles College of Chiropractic in early 1976 and was accepted for an interview. It seemed to go well but at the end of the interview, I had one question that had to be phrased as politely as possible: "I understand that there will be six years of academic work crammed into 4 years full time study to become a Doctor of Chiropractic. But do I have to take any more math?"

The Dean assured me, I had already met all the math requirements. That was all it took to say, "Goodbye, Cal Poly. Hello, Glendale, California." This decision was the best decision I ever made in my life. In September of 1976, I began medical school.

Day 2 on campus, I was face-to-foot with my cadaver. Every group of 3 to 4 students is assigned one. There's a specific cadaver room where all the dead bodies are dissected, muscle by muscle, nerve by nerve, artery by artery. The bodies are soaked in formaldehyde so they will last for an entire term of 18 weeks. The main rules in the cadaver room are not to eat in there and never wear anything that you want to wear in public again. Clothing picks up the smell of the cadavers and no detergent washes it out.

Let the Cadaver Capers Begin

Medical school is all-consuming. You eat, drink, and sleep with books, notes, and sometimes pieces of your class work. We would often stay in the anatomy dissection room until midnight, trying to perfect our surgical knowledge of the human body. Body part by body part, we would respectfully disassemble our cadavers right down to the smallest detail. With an exam every two weeks, there was always the threat of failing.

In fact, about 20 percent of the first term class did just that and never returned. The tests were the toughest I had ever taken and we had to virtually sleep in the dissection lab just to make sure we had learned our lessons.

Arnold was no exception to the rule. He was a bright Jewish boy who had been raised to excel. One night he was the last one in the anatomy lab. He decided to put in some extra study early in the morning at home before the exam. It seemed logical to take the cadaver's leg home since no one would be using it before the exam.

After six cups of coffee and 15 hours at school, this was fuzzy logic at best. He carefully wrapped the right leg of his cadaver in plastic, threw it in the back seat of his beat-up Volkswagen and headed home. This night, however, a taillight was out on his car. The police pulled him over and proceeded to write a ticket to this blurry-eyed student.

Arnold could grow a full beard by 11am so by 12 midnight under the cold stare of a policeman's flashlight, I'm sure he looked like the Son of Sam, a local and as of this night - uncaught serial killer.

As the flashlight scanned the back of the car, Arnold remembered the leg...

Within minutes, multiple police cars converged on the 'felon' with the remains of the dead and dismembered in his car. Helicopters circled overhead and for the next two hours Arnold was a crime scene!

The Dean of the School was brought down to the station, the body part was signed for and Arnold went home for an hour's sleep before his exam. The rest of us were never allowed in the dissection lab again after 6pm at night. Policy had changed and it would be the first of many changes created by the antics of our class.

Knowledge Equals Change

Over the next four years, it was imperative to master how the human body worked. The most important teacher was not on staff at the school; instead, he came to students via a weekend seminar. He completely changed the way I looked at my profession and healing in general. His name was Dr. George Goodheart, and he was a Detroit chiropractor who developed a system of chiropractic called Applied Kinesiology, or "AK" for short.

Goodheart asked us to constantly integrate what we knew as doctors, physiologists, nutritionists, and chiropractors. To positively affect the spine and its nerves which supply nerve flow to muscles, glands, and organs, we looked at diet, acupuncture meridians, blood supply, lymphatic circulation, and the spinal nerve supply all at once. The AK system was a more comprehensive method of achieving lasting correction to a problem. Goodheart's methods of balancing muscles allowed bones to stay in alignment and it was more specific and effective than standard manipulation alone. Reducing pain and increasing function to organs, glands, and joints all at the same time was a fantastic system, full of creativity and excitement. I could hardly wait to learn more.

Doctors Paul White, Dave Walther, and Bob Blaich, who wrote the initial textbooks in the field of Applied Kinesiology, were my mentors. Over the next four years, I studied over 200 hours with them. It also changed the way I studied in school. I didn't know it then, but this new philosophy would save my life years later and help uncountable others.

Squeezing a Relationship in Between Test-Cramming Sessions

As a single male in a primarily male class, I had surveyed the female situation without much hope – as you do. Within a few months I was drawn to M, a very bright Jewish girl from Brooklyn, NY who was part of my study group. Soon, we were inseparable.

She was the most gifted student and seemed always to get the highest marks in this competitive environment, much to the disdain of the Jewish males who considered academic excellence their domain.

M had been a philosophy major in University. She had turned down a Mensa invitation because she believed joining was an example of acting as an elitist. It was inspiring to see her study with a mind as tight and strong as an iron fist. She never lost sight of any detail, no matter how many there were or how minute it was.

The Business of Learning As a Medical Student

In chiropractic school, we soon realized that we had to study for content, not the tests. In the second term, we experienced a renaissance of learning because all the science background on the body was based on understanding it through systems. Learning was a group effort with so many notes to review and the constant pressure of exams. Often we would have 60 to 80 pages of notes to memorize 3 to 4 nights a week to ace the exams. With our small group of friends we carried the mantle of excellence late into many night cramming sessions. Ron, Dave, Fred, M, and myself, all excited and challenged to learn about the body.

For me, school was never easy. I was what you would call a "late bloomer." Finally, in the beginning of my second year of university at Humboldt State, I actually started to find myself in the context of academia. Broken homes and multiple negative primary school experiences had left more than a few holes in my learning skills and confidence. It was a big step to join the top students of the class in medical school and particularly one that was so competitive. I was proud of my As and Bs even though the rest of my group rarely got a lowly B at all. I found my stride and never looked back academically. Like a runner getting to the 6-minute mile pace of a marathon, the feet have the miles and the head has the drive.

As a natural athlete all my life, I found the hard work rewarding. Now with the help and guidance of M and my bright study group, I found my confidence in a system designed to destroy it! For the first time in my academic life, I felt at ease with learning. Now confident, I could focus on the bigger picture – real learning and not just the next test.

Before You Know It, You're Wearing the Graduation Cap

Upon leaving medical school, the first thing you want to do as a graduate and new doctor is start working; helping people with your newly licensed skills. Chiropractors are an odd lot in that all of us go straight out into the world starting our own practices from the ground up. There are no large hospitals or clinics to pay a wage. Many chiropractors who were great students fail in the business, lacking the confidence and skills to survive the market place.

I was lucky though, because I was also an "Applied Kinesiologist," skilled in the "AK system." I had spent my precious free weekends all through school taking outside seminars in AK, learning more. This gave M and I a little extra edge over other grads, and I felt that I had a full complement of skills to start my practice. The only question was where?

CHAPTER TWO
Colorado Country – Where It All Started

California where we graduated, the surf and sand seemed like an obvious place to open a practice but there was a problem. The State Board exams are only run twice a year and the Board takes another few months to review the results and mail the licenses, only if you passed! The time frame would be to graduate in December and maybe, by August, you could start practising! There had to be a better way.

Well there I was, still wet behind the ears, three weeks after graduation, wondering what life opportunities would present themselves. We took the Colorado State Board Exams and by January 7th, my results were in! M and I were two of the 48 percent that passed. We now had a license to print money... or so they said. Off we went in search of a home in the middle of a Colorado winter, with a canvas tent trailer on wheels – talk about optimistic!

Sometimes God Laughs at Our Plans

With $300 of graduation money in my pocket, the tiny Jeep and its heavy trailer full of medical books made its way over icy Wolf Creek Pass (elevation 10,857 feet), down into Gunnison Valley. And then it happened, the front wheel bearing decided to die in the -20 degree Fahrenheit temperature!

Through an amazing and almost inexplicable series of events, kind people took M and I in and welcomed us to the world of Gunnison. The dead wheel was fixed and with the help of a creative realtor, soon we bought a house to use for our practice – for no money down.

If You Build It, They Will Come

By April, I had built enough of the necessary items for practice. Lumber was made into chiropractic tables, benches, and even the dining room table. The front doors were opened with blisters on my hands. We called the practice Blue Spruce Chiropractic Arts. We set the fees and knew that the 3,000 inhabitants of that valley were unaware of how we were planning to change their lives and help them become healthy once again. Interest rates at that time were 24 percent and we had a mortgage to pay but, at $12 per office visit, we needed to see a lot of patients to make the house payment of $1100 a month.

And somehow it just happened; the money came when we needed it. We made our first payment and never looked back. Both of us had a good credit history and with the title of doctor in front of our names, the creative realtor Chuck was able to convince the bank we were a better gamble than the eminent foreclosure on the current owner of the house. Life was great. We both focused on our patients. We then realized that just 30 minutes up the road was Crested Butte and its ski area, which was a winter Mecca. Soon we found space and set up a "satellite clinic". Every other day we would drive from one practice to the other. Six days a week of work were all-consuming! With kinesiology skills, we quickly were taking care of the orthopedic problems, grumpy guts, parasite infections, blown out adrenals and blood sugar problems of a ski town and farming community alike. This gave us much-needed confirmation of the skills we had learned in and out of school.

Nothing But the Best for My Patients

Being knowledgeable in applied kinesiology chiropractic set our practice up for success and delivered great results with patients. After a year, it seemed second nature to prescribe vitamins, minerals, antioxidants, and enzymes for our patients. M and I were happy to be out of school, earning our own way, and utilizing everything we had been taught.

But life never stays the same. In early 1982, an official investigation was begun by a nutrition company we had started to rely on and use many of their products. They wanted to find out as to the nature and character of "the doctors" in Gunnison and why more nutritional supplements were being shipped to this practice than to all practices in the combined three adjoining states? Perhaps they thought that Dr. Stark was selling them to supermarkets or something that didn't meet their liking? These products are sold to doctors only, specifically chiropractors, as advanced and powerful formulations. At this time there was a renaissance in nutritional practices going on. Nutrition therapy with supplements was called "orthomolecular nutrition." The emphasis was on using high amounts and combinations of supplements to get drug-like immediate responses to illnesses, and it was working.

It turned out that the applied kinesiology teacher we had known since 1977, Dr. Paul White, owned the company that sold us the nutritional supplements. He quickly realized that we might actually be doing what he had instructed us to do in the classes he had taught. We were becoming local docs with a large following in the high country of Colorado, and our peers were beginning to take notice. Now the owner of the company we used wanted us to teach other doctors how to get the same amazing results on patients.

By late 1982, M and I had begun to lecture to our peers about how to use nutrition and the tools of physical diagnosis, in a holistic practice setting. Kansas, Texas and Colorado were just a few our weekend adventures on the lecture circuit. Our relationship was great the way it was and seemed perfect to both of us. Life was good, but Gunnison was, and continues to be, the coldest damn place in the continental United States. We were thinking about an easier life in California, one that was definitely warmer!

The Law of Attraction Comes Into Play

With the schedule of lectures and travel from remote Colorado, warmer climates appeared much more attractive to us. Because we had taken the California State Board Examinations in the summer of 1982, the test results were finally getting back to us, and having passed the California Board examination, options were opening up.

Life Decisions Can Be Quick but Results Slow

With the economy in recession, financial hardships in the smaller towns of Colorado were magnified. Once we made the decision to sell the practice and move to California, it took almost a year to finally hit the road. For three and a half years we pored out hearts into Blue Spruce Chiropractic Arts. It still remains to this day in Gunnison, as does its sign I hand-carved so long ago.

But now it was time to take a vacation, our first vacation ever. M had been to Europe just after undergrad school – I had never been off shore. We chose Europe and the time was the late summer of 1983. This vacation was our reward for the hard work – three-and-a-half years of six-days-per-week dedication to the Gunnison and Crested Butte practices.

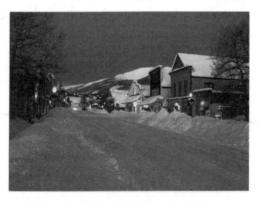

Crested Butte Colorado, where it all started!

CHAPTER THREE
California – Where It All Ended

Returning from Europe, we landed in La Jolla, California. Being originally from Santa Barbara, I knew that coastal towns were a ripe target for us to set up a new and more dynamic, holistic practice.

The friendships formed in chiropractic school are friendships for life. One of our friends we studied with in school, Fred, who put us up in his flash Malibu beachfront house when we first returned from Europe, helped us arrive at the name of our new clinic: Synergy Health Center.

The clinic was very successful and soon our workload necessitated that we put into place a management system that was based on 12-hour days. With a little financial planning, we were also able to make a system that was prosperous and successful. Life was good with a modest house on the hill overlooking the water. We had all the toys in the garage that we wanted. And best of all, we had happy patients.

We started to enjoy the good life with trips and excursions. A weekend in San Francisco, a seminar in Hawaii... Wow! In five short years, we were successful by all measures of our profession. Success was when you were published, lecturing, when you had happy patients, and when there was money in the bank.

On my birthday in 1986, M surprised me with tickets to New Zealand and Australia. Wow! I had been a surfer since the age of 10 and had always talked about going to these places, but now it was actually going to happen.

Not So Fast ... There Must Be Trouble

Just before we left on a holiday, I found a little bump on my testicle. I called Dave Simon, MD and friend, for a referral. He recommended consulting with an Urologist who then assured me that I had "epididymitis" (infection of the testicle) and with a course of antibiotics, it would resolve quickly.

It was now August 1986 and the surf was calling. Off we went to New Zealand. But despite the fact that I took the antibiotics, by the time I returned, the condition had not resolved. Not knowing what to expect, I put off an appointment for another six weeks after we returned from New Zealand. Finally, I went to see the Urologist in October.

The appointment was scheduled for a Thursday afternoon. During the Urologist's examination, his words struck fear in my heart. "It's probably cancerous and we must remove the testicle TODAY! The sun should never set on a testicle tumor," he said.

TODAY? This was happening too fast!

We compromised on the timing and I gained a few days. With surgery in the morning on Saturday, the deed was done by Saturday afternoon. I was soon at home with an icepack in my lap. The consensus was that all was safe. We would watch for signs of metastatic cancer. Over the next few months, I recuperated and did the medical monitoring necessary.

I was doing OKAY. Drifting back into the joys of full practise, I thought long and hard about the life I had made for myself.

The Good Life Had Been Earned and Was Rightfully Mine

When summer came I was overjoyed. The hectic pace of life in La Jolla could be counter balanced by trips to Palm Springs wallowing in the sun and swimming. I realized that I was at the zenith of my professional and personal life and all was good. The house on the hill, the toys, patients, and money validated that what I had worked so hard and long for was natural and destined.

What? More Trouble?

Knowledge about the body certainly does come in handy. On the second Tuesday in the August of 1987, it was time to investigate why my 6-week old cough wouldn't go away. It was a dry cough, the kind where nothing is spit up after coughing. It was possible that I had developed bronchitis.

Dr. Tain, a chiropractor and friend down the hall, had an X-ray machine and we casually took the X-ray. Chatting about this and that, Larry wandered over to the automatic processor as the film dropped into the slot. He held it up to the light.

When he turned, I could see his eyes had welled up with tears. I took the X-ray from him. I couldn't believe it was mine. It was the worst X-ray I had ever seen! Tumors were almost uncountable throughout the chest and heart spaces. **We both knew that I was a dead man walking.** Instinctively I comforted Dr. Tain with the words, **"I'm not dead yet!"**

Self-Diagnosis is Always Difficult

How could I have missed these signs? I had a persistent cough, one that lasted for a very long time. This is a bad sign as it indicates that healing isn't happening. My weight was actually much lower than I thought – I was down about 20 pounds. I don't know why I didn't notice that my clothes were looser. Hmmm.... My resting pulse was 137 – shit, I might only have a couple of weeks to live!

What Health Foundation Had I Stood On?

I walked back to the office and explained the situation to M, then went back to work for the rest of the day, spouting off about the righteous pathways to health to my patients. My words were hollow. My faith and foundation had been ripped apart in two minutes. What was I to do? I was so angry; everything I had worked so hard for was now worthless.

Things change. You adapt and learn how to deal with it, positive or negative.
It's a process. Bless it and learn to love it – it never stops!

Call In the Support Team

The first thing I did after talking to M was to call a friend and radiologist, Dr. Bielicki, to come to the office and confirm the findings.

Within a couple of hours he said that metastatic cancer was the only explanation; more than likely, it was testicular cancer that had spread to the lungs. He asked if I knew if the patient had a history of that. I confided that I was the patient and yes, about 11 months prior, I'd had surgery to remove a testicle.

Dr. Bielicki was on the inside of research and academia. He worked for the doctor who had written the definitive textbooks on bone radiology and knew who had the best reputations and medical acumen in San Diego. Only two met his high standards and criteria. Within a couple of hours, I had one of them, Dr. Stanton, on the phone. That was Tuesday.

Dr. Stanton was everything that Dennis said he was. Gracious and caring, he made time in his busy schedule to see me after hours in his downtown office. He was optimistic and said: "Chemo is the best option." After reviewing the slides of my surgery, he would have a more definitive answer.

Cancer often happens fast, and the next morning I was in the basement of the hospital in the pathology lab collecting my blood stained surgical slides from the pathologist, to deliver to Dr. Stanton's office. While looking at my blood on the slides, the whole situation became real. This was me! The few sutures and discomfort of the previous surgery were not a real representation of what the true reality had been this past 11 months. Now I had metastatic cancer throughout my lungs and chest. The truth was that I had a couple of weeks to live, at most! After delivering the slides on Wednesday morning, I went home to get my affairs in order. I was only 35 years old. The oncologist said he would meet with the Tumor Board at Scripps and we would meet on Monday. A Tumor Board is a group of oncologists that review all aspects of a patient's case and come to a conclusion about the best type of chemotherapy, surgery, or alternative protocol that will ensure the patient's quality of life. Hopefully, there would be a cure. A good doctor never tells the patient there is no hope, or you have X amount of time to live. Stanton was a good doctor; however, I was on the inside of the system and with 20 pounds missing in body weight and resting pulse of 137, I knew the end was coming fast, perhaps weeks or even days!

Easy to Let Fear Take Over When Things Take a Turn

Thursday morning was not good. I awoke with heavy lungs and a slight fever. While in bed the entire day, I wondered if my tumors were growing exponentially and taking over my body. The fight in my body was not going well. The fight in my head was not going well, either. This was it, not just it, but IT! The BIG ONE! How did I want to die? How did I want to be remembered?

I was dying. I sat up and meditated, breathing deeply and slowly for over an hour. The only hope I could have in natural therapy had long since vanished. Cancer therapy itself was as ghastly as the disease. I was trapped by fear. Was this my reality, a death wrought in fear, crying, and being sullen in the darkness of my own regrets? Whose choice was this anyway? I came to the profound conclusion that it was mine!

Dig for Strength Underneath the Fear

At that moment, the benediction of self-love, awareness, and gratitude overcame me. With what little strength I had, I let go, and accepted my death. It would be a calm and clear death, without fear, without remorse, without regret for a young lost life.

I chose to celebrate my path, the life lived and the wonderful relationships I had made along the way. You see, with a few days left to live, I came to understand that life is one day at a time.

When I had lost everything, I had found myself, my dignity, and my relationship with my own death. I had found everything of value to me, and it was "Stark".

Intuition helped me make decisions on how to live. Be present, clear, and careful with your words, emotions, and actions. Do not waste them on negative and dark moods – these really are a waste of time, time that you do not have as a luxury.

Make a Solid Vow to Yourself to Survive

I vowed there and then that if I somehow lived through this experience, I would dedicate my life to a better understanding of the causes of happiness and health in my own life. If I could, it would be an example for many and perhaps this painful lesson could be used to teach others how to avoid this ever happening.

Time Decisions are Always the Most Difficult

By Friday morning I was worse. M suggested we call Dr. Stanton, the oncologist, to give him an update on my state and find out if this was normal and expected? We were invited to come to the office within the hour. This was an ominous sign.

"You have the flu, Patterson, and we need to start chemo today. I am fairly certain the Tumor Board at Scripps Clinic would agree with the regime I am using. Are you comfortable with my starting prior to their approval?"

No anger here. This was a path to possible health, and it was one of the two left. I could do nothing, go home, perhaps develop pneumonia, and die, or start chemo with an optimistic view of a great outcome....

"Great," I said, "Let's do it." As the color drained from my face, my eyes became expressionless. All was as it should be.

Early Friday afternoon in Dr. Stanton's office, the IV was started and the Bleomycin, Vinblastine, and Cisplatin were titrated into my veins. I blessed the synthetic herbal therapy as they began;

I knew it was important not to resist. Also, it was important to embrace that which was the antithesis of my existence as an alternative healer. I let go and allowed the drugs to enter my body.

Within minutes of the chemotherapy starting, I could feel a difference, I looked at M across the room and she was crying but smiling. Cancer takes a toll on any relationship. She said the color had come back to my face and I looked better! I just smiled and said, "Of course, these are powerful herbs and the gods may have other plans for us that are yet to come."

I quickly received a confirmation about my decision. The chemotherapy cocktail was science's best effort at reproducing natural alkaloid drugs. When my color came back after the very first encounter, it was proof we were on the right track. American mandrake root, Madagascar periwinkle, and an ash of platinum were the basis of the chemo. These herbs were also a Vedic remedy for cancer and had been used over 3000 years. Scientific research had uncovered the ancient formula and improved upon it.

How fortunate!

My chemotherapy would be administered in a daily IV for five days, then one day per week for three weeks. Then the chemo treatment would begin again with the five days of constant IV. This was a cycle, which went on for 13 weeks. According to the oncologist, this is considered one of the two most difficult ones in all of chemotherapy.

Rapid Turnaround: Something Every Cancer Patient Wants

The response to chemotherapy was fantastic. Tumor mass was evaporating on the X-rays right before our eyes. Moreover, I was gaining weight! I had gained about 20 pounds.

Dr. Stanton was pleased with my progress. I had passed a milestone. He adjusted the chemo cocktail going into my body.

"Bill, I think I am going to beat this – there has to be a word for it."
"Apeori, Patterson," he said.

I was elated to hear that word and have to this day cherished the times in my life where effort and intent have yielded the desired fruit. It is very fortunate to have times like this in one's life.

On Monday after starting chemo, I called Marcia and Paul White, my AK teacher and owners of the nutrition company we had successfully used for the last five years. We had a nutraceutical program to build and it was mine.

Am I Ready to Graduate to Good Health Yet?

Thirteen weeks of chemo were finally over. However, my kidneys and liver were starting to shut down and my body could not take any more of the heavy synthetic drugs. The last X-rays were taken by Dr. Tain and unfortunately, the tumor mass was still present. It appeared that some of the tumors were resistant to the therapy. Dr. Stanton confirmed this, but what did it mean?

A lung specialist was called in for a consult, and between Dr. Stanton, the lung specialist, and myself, we laid the cards on the table. With the resection of 50 percent of each lung, the rest of the tumor mass could be removed. This was the surgical option. Without this, the surgeon assured me all the tumors would come back inside of six months.

Dr. Stanton, on the other hand, did not agree. He suggested my response to therapy had been good and perhaps we could wait and see. With monthly CT scans, the monitoring process would be exact and easier to follow than chest X-rays. I felt it was up to me to be the tiebreaker; as a doctor myself, my opinion was valid. Agreeing with the oncologist, we adopted the 'wait and see' approach.

Just Get Me on the Plane to Hawaii!

That decision not to cut out one half of each lung was made on a Thursday. On Friday, I was on a plane for Hawaii, and by Saturday, I was surfing the North Shore of Oahu. I'm sure I was the happiest baldheaded surfer that could ever be found! I had six months to live! As far as I knew it would take at least that long to kill me, according to the lung specialist!

Yes, the day I stopped chemotherapy, I went to Hawaii for a celebration of 13 weeks of therapy and while I could barely paddle out through the North Shore surf, that experience let me know I really was at my physical lowest of my entire life and needed to confront this when I returned to California.

Because chemotherapy is so hard on the body, your electrolytes (minerals) are often pushed to the extreme of physiological accommodation. This was my case as I paddled out against the surf trying not to be washed back over the coral reef, and it was the best motivation to paddle harder. My lats, the big swimming muscles, had been overdeveloped from twenty-five years in the pool and on the surfboard. I was a typical California surfer boy build, but under the influences of chemo, my best friends became my nightmare.

As I went under a wave, which was a second-nature experience for me, both of my lats cramped! My arms were pulled into my sides and I could not move as the six-foot wave pushed me down. My ability to hold my breath was also at an all-time low in my life, as I had just dissolved 12 of 18 tumors in there; I wondered to myself, was this it? Was I going to die by drowning? How freaking embarrassing!

Again, I came back to my new mantra "to let go", I relaxed instead of panicking and my arms slowly rose, allowing me to make it to the surface just as another wave hit. Tossed and turned, I went limp and let the wave push and pull my body apart, helping me stretch those lats out again. The only question was, did I have enough air in me to make it back to the surface? Somehow I did and made it out to the outside of the break where I sat for over 30 minutes before taking my wave to the shore. I was wiped out, but smiling.

In fact, during the time on chemo, there was a new mindset that sprung forth: There was work to be done when we came back from Hawaii. I bought a pair of running shoes and hit the road in San Diego. The problem was that I could only run about 200 meters before I became nauseous and heaved on the side of the road. Chemo was exacting its revenge. My resting VO2 max, a measure of oxygen uptake and efficiency, was below 20. This was average if you were in the intensive care unit! Yes, physical exercise was going to be a part of every day I lived. It did hurt – great!

I started running – but it was not easy. My body, which at one time had held hope for Olympic aspirations in Springboard diving, was now a train wreck of disjointed motion. For eight years I pounded the diving board perfecting "the dive" for the judges' approval; now I had to be my own judge and at the end of each day, I would run. Each step was slow and breathless. My coordination looked as if I had a hangover from a heavy night out even though I didn't drink... but I was above ground to feel it!

Look for Your Blessings and Focus on Them

I understood the spiritual significance of the situation; this was the last stand. Wasting days watching mindless television was not on the menu. Neither was wasting time on anything negative.

With a new set of exceptionally *low goals,* however, I blessed the fact I was alive and outdoors and could actually have the opportunity to even try to run. The body is a fantastic machine. With a little love and sunlight, it really responds. Within about three months, I was up to 40 minutes per day!

Create the Right Environment and Results May Follow

How cancer works at the cellular level is very complex. Cancer cells and healthy stem cells do not age and continue to multiply unendingly; this is part of the problem, and much research is devoted to halting this process in the cancer cells alone. All cancer cells divide in an anaerobic environment (with less oxygen in the tissues). Without oxygen, cancer cells extract sugar for fuel from the host (me) and multiply.

The job was to make my body an inhospitable place for cancer to live. As primitive as it may sound, if moving was aerobic and increased the oxygen in the tissues, it would be harder for the cancer to come back.

In the big picture, running every day was a very easy goal to achieve. It would take researchers another 15 years to prove that an hour of moderate exercise per day decreases cancer rates by 40 percent and improves cancer survival rates 40 percent also.

The next focus turned to the physical environment. It was clear that worldly possessions were valueless in my situation. They were actually a hindrance if you did not know why you had them in the first place. Difficult to give up? It took two years to sell all our personal belongings and hit the road. We had to get out of Southern California!

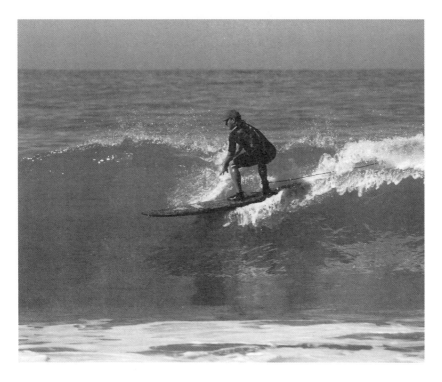

Kaikoura, NZ, a wave with no one around is a surfer's dream. Whatever the exercise – it must give you "juice" and surfing is one of my lifelong nourishing activities!

CHAPTER FOUR
New Zealand – You'll Be Right Mate!

The luxury of having six months to live is a very oddfeeling. When it's compared to the immediacy of the previous short-term prediction of two weeks, it's likehaving enough money in the bank to easily pay yourbills, with a little left over.

Here's a Question For You

What would you do with an extra $50,000? You can spend it on anything you want. Let's say that the world is offering you a chance to live any way you want. You can place value on anything or anyone any way you want. You can perhaps even travel. What would you do?

Too many choices can lead to a life filled with indecision. It was apparent I had little time to ponder the nature of the universe. My hand had been dealt.

Do the Opposite of What You've Done Before

Soon after chemo, I made the decision to set *lower goals* in my life. It seemed that the ego always had a way of expressing itself through the decisions made on a daily basis. Need a car? Then you must have the Mercedes. Need a motorcycle? It has to be the BMW. Just a chiropractor? No, you have to publish and lecture. It was all ego-based, but in my new humility and reality, these old ego needs were just not that important.

My new goal was maintaining the attitude that **every day above ground is a great day!** Period. True happiness suddenly was more attainable.

Draw Upon the Ancient Wisdom

In the mid 1980s, an explosion of Chinese culture was happening in the academic world. Ancient documents were being released to the Western world and translated for the first time. What I discovered was that Chinese medicine's deep underbelly was not obvious to the untrained. There was more to it than sticking needles in points to stop patients' pain. Thousands of years of esoteric knowledge, poetry and healing information was at hand and could be tapped into.

After reading more than a few books on the topic, I had found a friend in the ancient Taoist's decree:

"A man could not aspire to the enlightened realm, unless he lived 100 years. Only in this amount of time does a mere mortal have the ability to cultivate the appropriate understanding of the Tao (the way of life)."

That was it! If I was to live longer than six months, I must study immortality!

Chinese medicine is a fantastic system of healthcare. Over 3000 years of practice and observation had created a philosophical approach to health that was all-encompassing. Every facet of the diamond of life was reflected clearly and was in balance with all other tangibles.

Dr. George Goodheart, our applied kinesiology mentor, came a little closer to the mark as he had set the stage by intoning the fiveelement system as part of applied kinesiology many years before in my studies. By now in my life, it had been eight years of study of Chinese medicine and we had only scratched the surface. Intuition said there was more to learn and it had something to offer that might save my life.

Staying Free from Attachments is Part of the Answer

The "Living Tao" does not cling to life; any day is a good day to die. It was an interesting viewpoint to approach life without fear. On the other hand, I had to hope that what I did was creating a lasting immortality. This was what was called a Chinese paradox: Actions, which had lasting effects, were by nature, recreating karmic energy. Thus, whether it was murder or the act of not brushing your teeth, all action that was not clear and pure was recreating a response from the world directly back to the person who did the action. Buddhist doctrine told how hope and fear were the creators of samsara, the karmic cycle of birth and death. Living to make poor or improper choices and face the consequences became known as hell on earth or "Naraka!"

Eventually, the roots of modern Taoism led to my study of Buddhism. Finding a workable solution to the twin paradoxes was like a Rubik's Cube, and my life depended on the timely solution. I read more and more.

If living a long life was the key to understanding but clinging to a long life was suffering, how was one to reconcile the internal war of hope and fear? This was a question to ponder and it remained unanswered for another decade until an enlightened one set me straight.

An Insight From An Enlightened One

Over the last eight centuries, the Tibetan Lama, Khensur Thab-khey Rinpoche, would return to the world of suffering and patiently instruct those who would listen. He was ex-abbot of Drepung Gomang monastery in South India, and consecrated by His Holiness the Dalai Lama. At His Holiness' request, he came to New Zealand and created a center "Dedicated to Good Heart," Tashi Gomang Buddhist Centre, in Auckland. (It is interesting to me that "Dr. Goodheart" and the Center for "Good Heart" both are so important in my personal story many years later. Now I can see this. Wow!)

"Hope and fear always exist in the mind," he said. "The mind of awareness is constantly giving back hope and fear as illusions of reality." In complete or "enlightened awareness," one makes correct choices in life; therefore, bad or unfortunate results seldom occur. In this state, one has the "mind of awareness." This "mind of awareness" allows the ability to discriminate good from bad in today's world. The Lama believes that everything that happens to us comes from our black and white vision of what goes on around us.

He told me that my job in life was embracing Sunyata, which was insight into the emptiness of phenomena. "Emptiness is the key to freedom and liberation over the physical domain." I can still hear his words in my head through his interpreter Celia. This was the basis of the "Heart Sutra."

This was heavy stuff! However, so is life and death, and I noticed that he had my attention. I did not know how special this gift would become in my life. He had given me a great honor, an "Idam" (identity), a life path as seen by one who can see clearly the dharma of others.

Later in 1999, after the Lama's transition to the next world, his translator Celia said that the Idam was usually only given to monks after they had completed their training. I was again humbled. I cried that day, not with loss, but with comfort as I felt Rinpoche's compassionate energy on my shoulder. I knew it would always be there and for one of the first times in my life, I felt love, compassion, and acceptance of myself. It was just fine to be imperfect – that was the humanness of our birth. **Sincerity with purpose was what defined each person – this was the lesson.**

I now had an outline of how to live life and how to die. Both endings were acceptable. The circle from local doc with six months to live to Taoist-Buddhist had been completed. There was much work yet to do!

Why Did I Have Cancer? What Was Its Meaning?

There were still parts of my life that needed meaning. When one has cancer, the mind looks for reasons and justifications for the disease. Why does someone get cancer if they have the right body shape and are not obese in any way? Why does someone get cancer if they have a good diet, that is, one that is considered good by the standards of the day? If they have lived a clean life – one without alcohol or drugs, what causes cancer to start in the body? Even though my exercise regime was not regular, I could claim to be physically capable and perhaps even athletic. All this didn't make any sense at all. I should have been at low risk for cancer.

While reading the journals and researching the epidemiology of cancer and in particular, testicular cancer, I was immediately struck by the implication of radiation exposure for reproductive system cancers. The research suggested that my parents were exposed to radiation somehow, setting me up to express a damaged reproductive system.

If this was the case, then all I had to do was work long hours, increase my cortisol levels with the stress of medical school, my practice and the hectic life I had led for the last 15 years and whammo! The door was opened for the genes to go awry and multiply chaotically. Could this be the answer?

Is It Genetics that Causes Cancer ... or Something Else?

My father was in the Army and had been stationed in the South Pacific during World War II. I asked him directly if he had been exposed to any nuclear testing. He replied that he had not. However, he had been stationed on Guam and worked on the airfield as a fireman. It was his job to clean the planes when they returned from bombing runs. Guam was infamous for one plane, the Enola Gay. The plane, named after Col. Tibbet's mother, had dropped the atomic bomb on Hiroshima, Japan in 1945. When I asked Dad about it, he told me that everyone in the crew was very sick when they came back.

The plane itself was put to rest on one side of the field by itself. He said the plane was eerie because it made crackling noises as it just sat there. He did not think that was normal at all.

My father also stated he had a friend on the plane named "Cowboy." Dad was from Oklahoma and Cowboy was from Oklahoma or Texas. Within a few days, he lost track of him, as the crew was pretty sick; it was possible that Cowboy might have died.

After the war, my Dad paid a visit to Cowboy's mother. She said the army never told her how her son died or where; it was "classified" information.

My Father's Wartime Occupation Affected my Genes. Was There an Influence from Mom?

My mother had a much more compelling story.

When one forensically looks up a family tree, it's a wonder anyone is here at all. My mother was 28 years old when I was born. In her late 26th year, she and my father moved to the area of Rosemond, California, in the Mohave Desert, which is outside of Lancaster. My father had a job as a ranch manager.

Mom told a story about how they would go out to the desert in the cool evening twilight of the northern Mojave Desert to have picnics. Occasionally they would see very bright lights to the north in the direction of Nevada. This was between January and March of 1951.

During that time, Operation Ranger was in place and five nuclear bombs weighing 7100 pounds each were dropped on Frenchman's Flat, which is now part of the Nevada testing site. These were above ground tests dropped from a similar type of plane to the Enola Gay. The fallout drift spread hundreds of miles in the high atmosphere, only to be deposited on the fields of grazing dairy cows.

Like Chernobyl, it would be decades before the full extent of the radiation exposure would be known. As I asked more and more questions about my mother's history, it became clear she too was not only exposed, but also crippled by the fallout, in more ways than one.

I was conceived about a year after the nuclear tests between February and March 1952 and born in August. There had been a 7.5 earthquake towards the end of July centered close to where we were living. This might have explained why I arrived early at six and a half months.

A Pattern of Illness Spread Through Our Family

My sister Leslie was 7 years old when I was born. Like any young girl, she took immediate charge of mothering her new little brother. I was the next best thing to a real doll. Over the next year, she was always close and taking care of me, I only remember small glimpses of that time now. Tragedy was at hand. My sister Leslie lost her life, slowly and painfully, to leukemia during the next 18 months.

The illness and stress on the family was devastating. My mother suffered a nervous breakdown watching her child die before her very eyes. My father and mother were at the end of their relationship; they had no skills to overcome this. They parted ways and my mother, brother Ray and I moved to Santa Barbara to begin a new life; however, the footprint of radiation exposure was now stamped on our genes as we made a new home.

Putting more of the jigsaw pieces of my family picture together, about a decade later, I discovered that my mother had her thyroid removed. I asked if it was cancer. "No" she replied. The pathologist could not identify the cell type and while it was abnormal, it was not cancerous. This condition was commonplace with exposure to radiated milk and dairy products downwind of the nuclear testing. It was estimated that people could have had anywhere from 200 to 300 rads of exposure from the Nevada testing program that ended in the early '60s. One rad is the maximum yearly dose allowable for a human. Even today, we still say in radiation biology, "there is no allowable safe dosage of radiation" therefore, any dosage carries risk of developing cancer and must be weighed against the benefit to the patient with respect to the relative harm the procedure could create. Medical testing over-utilizes these modalities in my opinion, and in the opinion of many radiologists.

Taken together, my body was predisposed to some pretty clear risks to my health:

- my father's exposure in Guam from the Enola Gay
- my parents' exposure to the desert nuclear testing
- my sister's death from leukemia
- my mother's undiagnosed thyroid disease
- my testicular cancer

All these risks had occurred within a four-decade time frame, and it seemed fairly suspicious that I had developed cancer too.

Stopping the Cycle is Important to Eliminate Disease

As far as my physical environment was concerned, I came to the conclusion I was going nuclear-free and radiation-free. New Zealand became my focus as a first stop on the investigation of quality of life. I had a jogging habit to support!

If you had to leave town with only a backpack and no worldly possessions, could you do it? It would mean that you could put nothing in storage or in a garage. And, if you could, how would you go about getting rid of all that stuff that fills the cupboards of your home? This was the dilemma I faced with M as we had one garage sale after another. Rugs, blenders, pots and pans, and beds had to go. Then there were the bookcases and what should be done about those books? They had been collected from five years of undergrad school, five years of postgrad, and then of course, all the collections from the last eight years. It was not easy letting go, yet it seemed the only logical conclusion.

The hardest asset to eliminate though was the practice. Chiropractic or medical practices are sold every day. My practice was unique because we did not take insurance and we asked our patients to pay for their care as it was given. We did not have any accounts receivable and as strange as it sounds, it made it much more difficult to sell the practice.

The cash flow derived from old payments coming in while making the transition gives a sense of hope to the new doctor. We did have potential prospects that considered purchasing the practice but each new prospective doctor could not afford the practice. We were stuck in Del Mar and did not want to be there.

Eventually, a promising young doctor arrived and agreed on a price. We had to finance the deal; however, it allowed us to move forward with our plans. The first garage sale had been in early 1988. On April 1st, 1989, Del Mar was growing smaller in the rear view mirror. We had done it. With tickets in hand, we set off for New Zealand. It had taken over three years to return to the land of the Long White Cloud.

Thinking about the Past ...

After the 12-hour flight and the few extra hours it took us to get to the South Island and Christchurch, we were exhausted. Pre-booked into a hotel on Hagley Park, we crashed. The next morning when I awoke, I opened the door to find the newspaper and a glass bottle of milk on the doorstep. Wow, this takes me back 30 years in time when milk was in glass bottles with a little cream on top. The coffee was freeze-dried, and because we were on the other side of the world, it was simply like having an adventure! I put on my running shoes and surveyed the Park.

M and I walked the Park and began to plan our trip. We had three months in New Zealand to find out about this beautiful country.

Over the next week, we found a wee Mini in the paper to buy and with a copy of Frommer's guidebook, we set off for Akaroa and Banks Peninsula. At first view, Mt. Vernon Lodge was beautiful and understated and in the sun when we first saw it.

The owner, Hamish Johnston, was a dear man, a little younger than myself and by mid afternoon I was involved in moving hay into a barn and eating freshly made scones with hand churned butter from Fergi, the house cow. It felt surreal, transported back into a simpler time. Only a week before I was in my new car racing down an 8-lane freeway towards an office I did not want to be in.

Now I was talking about life and its meaning with people who actually had the time to do such things. What could I learn from them? How could this make me stronger? Even though I had increased my running up to about an hour per day, I could barely make it up the steep driveway at Mt. Vernon. There was more to physical conditioning than a pair of running shoes.

At this point, a most unexpected thing happened. After putting up the hay in the barn, Hamish said we looked pretty exhausted. I imagine we were pasty white with no muscle definition and little stamina. He suggested we take a couple of days and rest up in Charlie's Hut. We moved into a one-room sundrenched studio-hut with a potbelly stove, a writing table, bed, shower, hotplate and a porch that overlooked the Akaroa Harbour a mile below us. Other than the freeze-dried coffee, everything was perfect.

We came for only a day but over the three months in New Zealand, we would spend about four weeks total in Charlie's Hut. I began to write about my observations and noticed that my vitality and spirit started to regenerate. My eyes were drunk with fresh visions of beauty, and my soul had time to reflect. Another layer of health was starting to evolve.

As M had her philosophy background, we both agreed marriage was unnecessary and as we were both professionals, the thought of a family was not considered; now, post chemo, the thought of children was not a possibility. We did not feel remorse; we knew we had more to offer the world than our offspring. As we rested and talked in Charlie's Hut, a new exciting future started to be visible. Exactly what, we did not care as long as we were above ground to enjoy it.

CHAPTER FIVE
Humility – The Raft in the River of Life

I fell into a romantic love affair with New Zealand and with only six months to live, I wanted to enjoy myself. I knew enough to understand I may become medically unstable, but also realized that once again – I was face-to-face with making a decision that could change my entire life. Every morning I would look at my situation and decide how best to live the day! It was in one sense selfish and on the other, the only realistic thing to do. "Go fishing for myself!"

We had to return to the US to tidy up the last of our business, it seemed like a good idea to look around there, too. Even though our instincts said New Zealand was it – just migrate and live life.

When discovering my own roots, I found out that my mother's family came to the USA on the Mayflower in 1609. The US was as special for them as New Zealand now was for me. We bought a used Wesfalia Volkswagen camper in San Diego and took to the road in the summer of '89. It was an adventure. With New Zealand as our measuring stick, we went looking at the USA with new eyes. Community, freshness and a sense of belonging all seemed possible. Where was the place to call home in the US of A?

Over the next five months, we traveled through 32 states. From the forests of Washington to the coast of Maine, we looked closely at the structure of the country we had taken for granted all of our short years. At 38 years old, I did not really know if the cancer would just decide to grow back like a fungus over a neglected dish in the refrigerator. How do you decide when to make your stand and say, "This is it. I can live the rest of my days right here," without any regrets?

History Can Mean A Lot

Monticello was the home of Thomas Jefferson, the 3rd president of the United States. It was thought that he alone penned the Declaration of Independence. We walked through his home and read his memoirs; it was fascinating. This time period in history was centuries ahead of anything ever conceived in a government. As the Declaration was drafted, the inspired group of men in the continental Congress all knew the formation of a government was a pending death warrant on their heads if they did not succeed.

Was liberty worth the lives of family and community? History makes it clear that it was. My personal situation seemed just as large, but was I to renounce my country, rich in history, valor, and character? It seemed like an overwhelming task. More information was needed, on to John Adams' home we went. The relationship between Adams and Jefferson was tumultuous, to say the least. Their ideals were at opposite ends of the spectrum. However, the tolerance, built into the new Constitution, became a standard by which all men could measure freedom. The separation of church and state was absolute in Jefferson's eyes, while a country "under God" was assured that the "right god" was no longer an issue. Personal freedom was pragmatic – choose what ye will and free will to all men.

It was in "stark" contrast to the Cathedral in The Square in Christchurch and most other New Zealand towns and cities. The Royals and the Anglican Church all seemed opposed to the concept of personal freedom, let alone Jefferson's assertion that all men are created equal. This was good stuff. I was lost in my head and immersed in the romance of Colonial America. A wake-up call was necessary; the universe would soon provide it directly and forcefully. There was one more President's home to visit.

General George Washington became the 1st President of the United States. The Congress of those 13 colonies did not hesitate to put a reluctant Washington into a position of power, which was so far, loosely designed. As history recorded, the term of the presidency was not set as it is now. The idea of noble and patriarchal leadership was the only known method of government. Feudal and with subordinate taxpayers, the system was not good enough. The US, from the time of the revolution, only existed with a militia, held together by Washington's character and strength. The Articles of Confederation were in place, but the formation of a central government was yet to be accomplished. A new declaration demanding a different standard had yet to be written.

A government with a presiding President and representative Congress would be formed. The British were defeated in Boston in 1776; the last major victory in Yorktown 1781 closed the colonial door however, it would take until 1789 before the present constitution was in place replacing the Articles of Confederation. Ending with two 4-year terms as President, Washington's desire to keep the US out of foreign wars was ratified by the Proclamation of Neutrality in his last year in office. No longer would the US be drawn into conflict. The tenured general knew that the country needed time to build its infrastructure if it was to survive. How things have changed in just over 200 years.

Becoming a Crime Victim Changes One's Perspective

As I returned back to the Camper from George's Library at Mt. Vernon, my heart sank. The car door was open and broken glass lay on the ground on the driver's side. My property had been violated! We had been robbed! While we had renounced all of our worldly possessions, four months on the road meant we had accumulated a few necessities.

The surfboard that was used on the waves of Lake Michigan was still on the roof, and many books and even a laptop computer were stored away in the camper. We were very lucky. Here we were at the house of the 1st President of the United States, in clear view of hundreds of people and the car had been broken into. Was nothing sacred? In fact, it was not. The thieves hadn't taken much, but with an unsecured car, we could not stay in the Washington area. We left and headed north up the eastern seaboard, but in our hearts we knew the US was no longer our home.

Practising Detachment and Searching for More Meaning

At this time, my daily running habit had already been underway for over two years. I looked healthy, yet I did not feel even close to vibrant. Traveling at a leisurely pace, I would read more of my Taoist books every day and settle into contemplation about the meaning of what I was reading. The concept of detachment was the aim if one was to become an immortal according to the ancients. Detaching from worldly possessions had taken a couple of years, but more baggage remained between my ears. Ego attaches meaning to everything; it is the basis of how everyone operates. We place a value on almost everything in our world by how we perceive it – some would suggest with ego.

That is where the real problem lies – in the process of perception. Hot and cold, and light and dark are two dualities similar to yin and yang. If you are concerned about monsters in the dark, you give a graded or shaded meaning to the word dark over light. All the experiences in your life accumulate to refine the way you look at life. These experiences become filters through which you look at life and they define objects, feelings, and meanings of everything that happens in the future. The filters are very personal to you.

For instance, if you have skin cancer, sunlight has a different meaning for you than for me. In fact, the more I looked at how I thought and what I thought, the more it became clear that the color I saw around me in my life was in fact, a figment of my own imagination. It was a startling revelation – I was living in my own dream and trying to sell it to the rest of the world... Like other people, I only had one "learned" set of experiences to judge my life and interactions to this life with. Hmmm, I need new experiences.

The key word was "revolution," as I took stock of the works of Thomas Jefferson. He was a renaissance man in every sense of the definition::author, statesman, botanist, cartographer, meteorologist, and architect who could read and write six languages. Was he living a dream, too? I looked deeply into the meaning of a man's existence, specifically my existence. What would be my legacy? What dream was I to live each and every day? Who do you please on a daily basis that has a different agenda than yours, and why do you do it?

Clarity of purpose may be strangled by rhetoric. Did I have a need to live? Was it just greed that made me want to live another day? I mean, living is the objective of life, but no one said it had to be a quality existence, did they? Having additional days in life equals a more valuable life, or does it? I felt the "Taoist Immortals" again had proven their value with the pragmatic creed of longevity. In between the martial arts, meditation, and stringent diets, these ancient Chinese Adepts' practices are called the "humor of longevity. "

There's a saying that has stuck with me from that time. "One is just human and you must master all forms of human existence (gain personal experiences); only with mastery can you understand they have no value!" That's what the Chinese believe.

They went on to clearly state, "This will take about 100 years and will fill up your life with meaning enough to allow you to understand the Tao." It is the way of life that leads us – not us who leads the life. I started to understand deeply; I did not have a choice about my journey, it was either in the living world or it was not. Humility now presided over ego. As difficult as the task seemed, there was a place for my own renaissance over the dream. All I had to do was embrace the way of life and not struggle with the interpretation from the ego. If I could clearly see what was worth living for and put effort in that direction, then it would be easy to let go of the practices that conflicted my life.

All these thoughts were streaming through my head as I sat behind the wheel of my Volkswagen and made my way back towards California. It was a direct route back and we were being pulled Down Under.

Starting Each Day with a Purpose

With a new found sense of humility, I began each and every day with a purpose. I was part of a precious life, allowed to live another day. All that I did had implications and consequences on the world. My job: understand how significant these actions were! In the context of "the self," the actions are fairly easy: eat right, exercise, take my vitamins, and meditate every day to have a strong body as a base of experience, a base of awareness. Relating to others or the rest of the world, it was a little more obscure.

To the best of my ability, I had to work to master that which was in front of me. I was humbled again by the fantastic opportunity that every day brought to learn, live, love, and have reverence for the process. This was the life I wanted more of, but at the time I was working on detaching from that need, as I wanted it!

Again the humor of the Chinese was apparent. Lost in the essence of human existence, it becomes apparent that one has to listen to his or her own destiny, *master the tasks seen as important, and be respectful of the efforts of others who must do the exact same thing as you do each day.*

The Meaning of Tradition

When bowing to another in the Buddhist tradition, you place your hands together and bow three times. First you bow with hands over your forehead, next over your throat and lastly over your heart. This is a conscious acknowledgement to the person in front of you of three important understandings.

- You are saying in the form of formal prostration, I bow and salute who you have been before me in the past, and all that you have gone through to be that person.

- I bow and salute who you are now; the struggle and liberation you experience on a daily basis.

- I bow and salute who you will become as a person and fellow traveler in the sea of life.

Doing this creates humility. It becomes apparent that everyone is in the process of doing exactly what they are meant to be doing at any one time. It is all perfect. LIFE IS A GIFT. RESPECT IT.

When I Looked, Life Was a Series of Awakenings

We had driven over 25,000 miles to find America. The journey had awakened a deep-seated connection not only to the United States of America, but also to the world. It did not really matter if we stayed in the US, just if we stayed on the planet. This was the pragmatic discriminating awareness the ancients were alluding to. Now what location does my heart call me to? Again, the ego would cloud the perceptions and our course would be pulled and tossed about. We were on our way to... Australia! New Zealand was nice, but Australia was bigger and more economically secure. We were on a "walkabout," which is a traditional Aboriginal walk of independence into the country. We understood the US held no future for us.

Dr. DeVoy had come to the US and visited our clinic in La Jolla, trying to glean some experience from our use of the advanced chiropractic techniques on our patients. We had met him at seminars in California and in Hawaii, and on that fateful trip with a bump on my testicle, he was as eloquent and gracious as he was on our first meeting in Australia. On that visit, I had met many of his professional associates in Sydney. They were all very professional and liberal in their views; additionally, they exuded a vibrancy not seen in California.

It seemed as if Australia was the Promised Land for alternative medicine. Although I was not interested in practicing again, it was comforting to know this existed. Australia was to us, at this time, a big New Zealand. We arrived in Sydney, bought a car and went looking for our place. We had decided to emigrate to Australia and filed our applications before leaving the United States.

After traveling the States for five months, we were seasoned in the art of investigation; yet Australia was fascinating and the wildlife was teeming with diversity, the likes of which we had never seen. We were in awe of the "Lucky Country" as it was called. We had arrived in October, and began traveling north from Sydney. We made our way to Cairns, in the Northern Territory, then we traveled all the way west across the country to Perth. Sadly, we were devastated by what we found.

As we had learned in the US, it is a land not made just of dirt, but of the people who live there. During our trip through rural Australia, we came face to face with the Aboriginals. As we learned about their history and in particular the history of the invasion of the "white fellas," we could see the Native American Indian plight all over again. Unlike the sheltered parts of the US where we had lived, racism was alive and well across Australia. The average person we sat down with to talk to was not even aware of their attitudes and this made it both forgivable and revolting at the same time.

M's grandparents had many friends around the house when she was growing up who bore the tattoo on their wrists from the concentration camps in Germany and Poland; she knew discrimination first hand. I could see this in her eyes. Professional friends in the city had been cosmopolitan in their views; the contrast was unacceptable. Around Christmas time in Perth, we sold the car and bought tickets back to Christchurch. We were going home!

We stopped at the "dairy," a little market in Akaroa for some groceries before we went up the hill to Mt. Vernon. We hadn't been in the store for almost 10 months, yet the owners greeted us by name and asked what we had been up to. The sense of belonging was overwhelming, and parking up the familiar drive, we settled into Charlie's Hut again.

Cultural Differences and Lifestyle Differences

Later in the month I met a young surfer on the West Coast. I told him I had lived on a hill very much like the one behind the surf break we were surfing and that you couldn't see the hill itself because it was completely covered with houses. He thought that was outrageous and said he had seen some pictures like that on television.

What he could not fathom was "shopping." I told him when I went to the "supermarket" for food, the store was as large as 10 shops in Greymouth put together, and in a year of shopping there two or three times per week, I never saw a person I knew, let alone someone who knew my name. To this boy who had grown up in a community that knew him, his family, and his history in the blink of an eye, it was bewildering why or how someone could live in such isolated circumstances. I told him it was because we could drive a Mercedes and eat out a lot.

"Why would you do that when there is such good food at home?"

"That's exactly why I'm here!" I replied. The memories all came flooding back to me as we went to sleep on the hill overlooking Akaroa and its bay harbor.

Still Alive and Kicking Means Start Planning; Life's Not Over Yet

After three years, I was still alive and it appeared I might have another six months to live. There was no sign of cancer on my X-rays, and I was in remission. The long and hard-fought fight had taken us around the world. We had studied many cultures and learned much about the history and people we encountered. Our final decision was to stay in New Zealand! We felt our choice was supreme and proceeded to apply for residency, but had still not heard a word from Australian immigration.

The humility we felt at the opportunity in front of us when we applied for residency was suddenly steeped in fear; what if we were not allowed to stay? In our minds, we could not return to the US or Australia, and we did not want to leave New Zealand!

Carefully, we crafted our applications. I had to take and pass the New Zealand Chiropractic Boards. I hadn't taken a board exam in close to eight years, yet everything was riding on my success. A half-day of written exams was followed by a practical interview where I could be asked any question about any subject. It was a difficult test, thorough and comprehensive, and many did not make it. I was fortunate and received high marks in most areas. With this hurdle overcome, I now had a license and could apply for residency. Unlike my first license to "print money," this one represented a "license to live!" Now, I needed a job.

It was time to go back to the West Coast and the good Dr. Reiderer, a Swiss born, Canadian-trained chiropractor who had settled in the small town of Greymouth. We had met in Akaroa at Mt. Vernon on the first trip, and visited him and his family when we traveled to his side of the island. As was the way with most Swiss people, you will always find a set of "Lederhosen" in the closet; they take national pride with them wherever they go. Stephen and Corrine were no exception. With three beautiful young children, they had settled into an ideal lifestyle a couple of years earlier. They had freshly baked bread every morning, chooks (chickens) in the garden, and a warm fire in a kitchen filled with relics of their homeland. The children were being raised to be bi-lingual, not tri-lingual like their parents, and all was good. We came to terms about employment. A letter was written to Immigration asking for my skills, and we sat back and waited for the wheels of progress to turn. We wanted to settle down and stop traveling for a while. We needed to nest.

The sale of the practice in La Jolla, the two trips to New Zealand, and travel throughout the USA and lastly Australia had cemented our commitment to a life of health and comfort. We thought we had our priorities just about right. We just needed the New Zealand government to agree. On a 3-month visa, which had been extended once, we were running out of time. We would have to leave the country if the passports did not come in the mail soon. Finally, on the last day before we were supposed to leave, it was obvious we had to do something, so we drove to the Christchurch Immigration service.

Something Had to Happen Quickly

Without an interview or appointment, I casually walked up to the counter and explained I had traveled from out of town and thought I would save the government some courier money by personally picking up my passport and my new resident's visa. The young clerk told me to take a seat while she checked on the progress of the application. It seemed like hours. If we were declined residency, we would have to be on a plane the very next day. Everything was still in Akaroa, and although we didn't own a lot of belongings, it would be a logistical nightmare.

"Dr. Stark," a voice said. I went up to the counter and the clerk said, "Here you go..." and handed us our passports.

Had our passports been declined? Had she just misunderstood, retrieved the passports and halted the application process? In the blink of an eye she was gone and we just stood there for a frozen moment and looked at each other in disbelief. I then decided to open the passport. There, in the back was an official document with these words below:

"PERMANENT RETURNING RESIDENT'S VISA" We were in. We made it home!

A new phase of our life was beginning. We had learned much theory, read many books, traveled great distances, and now had a homeland to live in. How were we going to apply this knowledge and put it into practice day by day? How were we going to take our health to the next level? No one had written that book yet. We had to use our intuition and educated guesses about the best way to stay on the planet. This was another new adventure. Patience and compassion are very similar. Both require a concerted effort to achieve. We moved away from the hammering southerlies to Nelson at the top and warmest part of the South Island. It was a warmer microclimate with a small community of liberal-minded people, and Nelson felt like home.

The raft of ideas and practices that we had clung to on the last three landmasses were now moving us from the river of life to the ocean of life. The turbulence seemed to fade away as we became more focused on the methods and practices we had collected. Compassion was now used on ourselves. We could live freely and without the need to work so the ideal lifestyle was possible.

What exactly was the perfect lifestyle? What was the perfect life and why did it have to be perfect anyway? This was going to be fun now that the frustration of choice had opened the door of compassion. Not so much to others, but to ourselves; we were still clinging to excellence as a form of ego, not a measure of mastery.

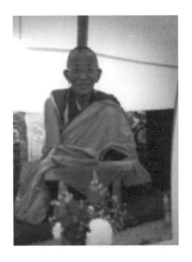

Khensur Thabkhey Rempoche, (1927 – 1999)

"SMILE; you're above ground!
You have so much to be thankful
for – it is a human and precious
birth you were given, honor it with dignity."

CHAPTER SIX
The Ocean of Compassion and the Agony of Ecstasy

Having moved into a furnished apartment overlooking the city of Nelson, we were spoiled. The Banks Peninsula with the small town of Akaroa is about the size of San Diego, but with perhaps 2000 people spread evenly over the entire area. It is rural, to say the least.

Nelson, on the other hand, is the hub of shipping, commerce, and cultural life for the northern part of the South Island. The town has a population of 5000 but provides services for about 50,000 provincial inhabitants. The contrast from the 3 million in San Diego was quite refreshing.

What would you do on a daily basis if you did not have to work? How would you spend your time? I had learned a few things in the years since that day my life suddenly changed. Now I had the opportunity to use what I had learned and sculpt my masterpiece lifestyle. Where to begin was the question.

I had continued to study health, starting from scratch with soil chemistry and farming practices. New Zealand was a perfect place to see it all in action; farmers were everywhere, and very switched on about the practises on their land that promoted life. I had many discussions about short-term gain verses long-term stability and sustainability. The farmers were pragmatic and caught in the same cycle that city people were stuck in – both had mortgages to the bank.

Life is Straightforward on a Farm

On the farm, production is everything; a farmer might only take stock to market a couple of times a year, so cash flow depended on how much you could get for each "stock unit" per acre of farmland. This seemed straightforward, but to make a profit, service the bank, and feed the family, it took hard work and constant diligence. The weather could devastate your profits for the year by delivering a late snow. Without enough grass to feed your animals, financial stress could easily be created.

Thankfully, the farmers had help from the petrochemical industry. It was easier to force the grass to grow when you applied the "super phosphates" on a regular basis. Lending extra money for chemicals was a sure thing for the bank. The bank managers were usually farmers themselves and were an integral part of the farmer's life and business strategy. The problem was that the extra amount of stock you could run was barely enough to offset the cost of the chemicals. At the end of the day, you had to put the chemicals on the property to maintain high numbers of stock units so you could service your mortgage and keep the bank manager happy.

The "Super Phos" was akin to junk food in humans for animals. High acid minerals would push the alkaline-producing clovers; yet reduce the overall mineral content of the grass by 200-300%. Thus, animals would be stressed, have lower rates of reproduction, and higher rates of infection, including parasite infestation. That's when the pharmaceuticals could come to the rescue with increased frequency of drugs to get the animals to market with the higher dollar cost, in addition to a depleted and lesser animal.

Occasionally, I would find organic farmers who raised sheep, cattle or dairy cows without the aid of chemicals. We would talk at length about the problems of the herd and how difficult it was considered to find real sustainability. When the chemicals were not used on the land, the stock units could not be sustained at the previously high levels but the birth rate per animal increased in the first season. Most animals like sheep and cows are capable of twins, especially sheep. Starting with a hundred sheep, in theory you could produce 200 lambs. The ratio is usually more like 1.3 per ewe and that ratio is tracked as an indicator of herd health and vitality.

Without the expense of the chemicals on the grass or in the animal, a common pattern that occurred after five years was found amongst the farmers' herds. Herds were very disease-resistant, and lambing and calving rates were the highest ever seen by these farmers (2 lambs per ewe or more). Costs were down. Even with the lower stock units, profits were up convincingly. Critically, farmers were looking after soil health by using natural products. They knew the ability of the soil to hold water was important and it was all about the roots, fungus, and timing of the paddocks.

They also learned that nutrient content was important. The more varied the grass was on the land, the deeper the water would soak in, enabling the bacteria and their fungus in the soil to work more efficiently, creating a drought-proof, healthy, "mixed salad" for the animals with diverse mineral content. While organic farming would take another 20 years to really catch on, there was more to this "sustainable farming practice" than people were ready to give credit to. Even the government had a "sustainable lifestyle" attitude that would later be known as the "Nanny State," where everyone would be taken care of by the State if things got tough.

Cultural Differences Dictate a Lot of Attitudes

In cities in the US and in New Zealand, most people had a mortgage. The beauty about Nelson was that houses were more affordable and people seemed less concerned about driving new cars. We still had a Mini at this time. The closest shopping mall was in Christchurch, five hours away. Yet people had to go to work to service their mortgage, so life was directed again by their relationship to their bank.

Unlike the US, in New Zealand, if you could not pay your loan, the bank would just forward you some funds to tide you over. This was done in the form of an "overdraft." I discovered that many people used this facility and the banks made a killing. As a result, folks could put off the realities of their existence and consume a little more than they might have. It was like the farmer getting a little more grass off the land than he might have with the use of the chemicals. People were tied to the bank whether they liked it or not.

What Causes Mental Stress for One Person is Different in Another

The interesting thing was that most New Zealanders I talked to were not too upset about this at all. It never got in the way of vacations, and no one ever slept on the street. The socialized structure of the government was the ultimate middle class; if you couldn't pay, the government would always help you out for a while. With this easy life, people did not need to push hard for production and the backyard garden was declining in popularity.

Still, about half the houses on our street in Nelson had workable gardens compared to zero in Del Mar, California. Veggies were bought at the "veggie shop" and meat from the local butcher. Every corner seemed to have them available. I could not remember the last time I had been to one in San Diego! The veggies had mud on them and had been harvested the day before.

In the US, the average veggie spends 14 to 28 days in transit from field to mouth. If a veggie loses up to 50 percent of its vitamin content each day after picking you can do the math as to which might be the better animal on the farm, so to speak.

At this time in the early 90s, the Kiwis numbered a little over 3 million. What was fascinating was the vitality of the country as a whole. The entire population of New Zealand could fit into San Diego County! Yet, the country held 50 percent of the world records in Masters Track and Field! Maybe the stock units could be counted in different ways when it came to farming a healthy herd of people? They could "punch above their weight" as was often said (underdogs that rarely lost). In Rugby – the national game – England, with a population of tens of millions, had only managed to beat New Zealand a few times in the last 90 years!

The Search for Balance

My study of the Tao had shown me all things must be repaid. Yin and Yang must balance. We had the opportunity to live for the first time in our lives debt-free, with unlimited time (six months), and only our imagination to restrain us. What a gift! How would we maintain balance? Most people could not relate to this amount of freedom; it's a life's dream to be unencumbered by a mortgage or constant duties that dictate what you do on a weekly, monthly, and yearly basis. We were different. We knew things, or did we?

When truly honest, you realise how much pain it takes to make you move. The cattle prod on the farm quickly moves a stubborn cow, but what does it take to quickly move you, or me? The cattle prod is a lot of energy and pain packed into a very small unit of time. If you or I experienced a cattle prod, we would have a graphic and vivid memory of the event for quite some time, perhaps years! It is the intensity of an event in time that gives it meaning. Cancer had been my cattle prod; you might ask yourself what yours have been?

Rules of Life

Order must have disorder. What is known must have an unknown component and certainty must have uncertainty. The relative world of work, shop, sleep, and work again must have a weekend with a promise of the unknown and fun in order to happen. These are the rules of the game of life on a very basic level. If we had all the freedom in the world, yet did not understand the rules, what good would it be?

We realized now that the bank does not make the rules of life and we could do anything we wanted, we just had to design it. Yes, this is anarchy if you're looking at it from the bank's perspective.

Most people we met conformed to rules that they did not make, in a system they would never design, and usually in a place they would never choose to live. It had taken me close to 40 years to understand I was living in an artificial, mentally constructed world without conscious understanding of its implications in my life. I felt a little jaded. How was I supposed to act without "those rules"? What would happen without them?

I felt as if the keys to the Lamborghini had just been given to a 16-year-old. Fantastic, exciting, and dangerous! I could now construct the perfect life, but perhaps perfect was the wrong word? I mean, I still had to consider detachment and everything else...

CHAPTER SEVEN

Gratitude – A Reason to Live Better, Longer, and Stronger

Compassion is the realization that your actions have implications for the well being of others. With this understanding, a decision can be made to choose that which will benefit those in need. In the Buddhist tradition, this is called the Bodhisattva Vow. You take it for the sake of all sentient beings (those who have not found their way to happiness or liberation) and choose to return to the land of struggle and toil for the sake of helping others, even though you could live forever in paradise. This is a very significant realization and statement for one to make. Return to the real world and work harder... it sustains a life compassionate with actions for others because you can and see the dilemma. What is the value of paradise if there are still others suffering? Merely, the illusion of paradise I say, as paradise does not segregate – everyone gets in.

It would be a few more years before I took my personal vows. The Universe was already asking me the question loud and clear... *"Kid, what are you going to do with your life?"* Wouldn't you feel just a little guilty about the fact you are indulging in only self-serving actions? The "Work Police" could come around the corner at any moment! I thought about my situation. I started working at about 12 years of age, finished med school at 28, and six years later I was still working seven days a week when cancer came to teach me a lesson. After a couple more years of work, I abandoned "work" – as I knew it – to essentially go on a quest! I find what I am looking for and yikes, I then have to construct the perfect life, or deconstruct my values and worldview. Poor me?

In reality, it was not that difficult, but more like putting a foot into a warm bath that was just right. Nelson felt good, and the body just followed along. Reconnecting to "things" was a little odd. Having an entire apartment to ourselves for the first time in two years was a conscious decision that made us appreciate just how little we needed materially to make life work. Now our needs were "stark" in comparison to the house on the hill in Del Mar.

Re-Invent a New Life

I had a feeling that what I had to do could only be done once. It had to be done with reverence. The new lifestyle in Nelson needed a strong base. Balance was necessary to ensure that my fragile body would last the entire six months; the imaginary amount of time it would take to die if all things went wrong and the cancer came back.

I felt that it could work out and made a list of the perfect lifestyle:

- Join a gym, something we had never done before.

- Continue in the internal arts of meditation. This aspect of life was taking on new depths as the internal alchemies were experienced from the inside out.

- Ponder about passion. What was passion, anyway? I felt that it was pivotal to longevity as an emotion and had many positive side effects. I had once had passion for architecture – could I actually experience passion again?

- A reading list, long and interesting.

- Cooking needed to be explored in our new kitchen and a garden planted.

And so life became the gym on a daily basis, excellent food, books, and a time to nest. Life was good in Nelson. M and I were getting stronger, both mentally and physically. We started some design classes at the local Polytechnic and settled in. The renaissance had begun in full. Though we were not in the league of the peanut farmer from Georgia (Jimmy Carter, President, humanitarian, farmer, nuclear physicist), we felt proud of our new life. There was a satisfaction from establishing a new lifestyle on our own without the help or vision of those who had done it before. Actually, we did not know anyone that had accomplished our goals. There were no mentors and in fact, another decade would pass before I understood the significance of having mentors.

One unexpected spin-off of our interaction in the Nelson area was that we were meeting people while doing activities. This social interaction was different. No longer was I called "Dr. Stark." Now the interaction was simple – how good was your project in design? How much could you bench press? How much are you laughing on a daily basis? It was honestly the first time I felt accepted for who I was as a person, not who I was trained to be as a professional. We had community for the first time. And, I also became a Godfather to Vinnie!

Lifestyle. The word itself denotes some panache, a little art-like flair, which adds fun to "life." We understood, as doctors and now people, that we are living gratefully in the world, that it took balance, planning, and oddly, spontaneity to keep the animal alive. This mental construct was the basis for exploring joy and happiness over the next five years in Nelson. This was a clue to what healthy people do, and the idea, though fleeting at first, stayed with me.

Mike was a second-degree black belt in the Okinawan style of Bushin Ryu Karate. (He is now a 7th dan). He was a couple of years younger and about the same size physically. He worked as a personal trainer at the local gym we belonged to and taught his own karate classes in a church hall four times per week. Mike suggested I come to a few karate classes to see if I might like them. It was not long before I had the full kit, white belt and all. With aerobics classes, weight lifting and yoga, the Karate made for a full physical schedule as the renaissance marched on. With the change in my physical program, I passed another milestone.

It had been a little more than two years since I stopped chemotherapy. The massive implosion of tumors in my lung cavities had left scar tissue, which caused a deep aching pain that migrated to my ribs at different points. This was disconcerting as it always felt like the cancer was returning. I felt it wasn't, but how could I be sure? I had a fool for a patient before, and that was me.

My theory was that the scar tissue would be stretched during the course of normal activity. When it broke, inflammation would be part of the repair process and I would have the sensation of the aching pain from the swelling. There was a gnawing doubt about this, but after about six weeks in the gym I had notched up the bench press and loaded the thoracic cavity in a way that had not been done since my college days. The pain was gone! Real strength was returning for the first time in a decade and life was interesting. Retirement was fantastic!

The Monks Had It Right

It was about this time I really began to get my head into Taoist philosophy. The longevity aspects of the formal training of monks made perfect sense. In the last millennia the training had been refined to a high degree with every question about the human body's needs and how to care for it answered, a pragmatic detachment to life or death was the bottom line against which all was measured. It set up the view of the world for the master. It gave me a foothold, as I did not have a living mentor or map showing me how to proceed.

The goal was to live another six months. A loose system of exercise, diet, and study had begun in earnest and I now had friends with historical accounts of monastic life. Yet the Chinese paradox was that I could not cling to the outcome. I had to let go and live each day; each moment needed clarity, conviction, and passion.

My first understanding of Chinese medicine was in medical school almost 14 years earlier. Now the dissection of the rich world of ancient China gave color and meaning to the formulae I had used in the treatment of my patients. It was essential to know the acupuncture meridian system to practise meditation, martial arts, and how to eat correctly. Everything has a purpose, life is never a system of compartments; life is whole and connected. What one did in the kitchen allowed martial arts abilities to be purely expressed, which then allowed full mental faculty for the meditation practice.

Classical Chinese education would require other involvements if one were to be an "Immortal." Music, poetry, calligraphy, martial arts of many styles, and even the bedroom arts were all considered areas necessary to master. My retirement did not have enough hours in the day. It was humbling to realise how much I did not know and how much existed at such a detailed and exacting level. The lesson was to learn and master all, and then find it wasn't necessary in the first place. The process takes about 100 years according to the Taoists.

Nelson provided a stable environment for in-depth study, punctuated with travel to Australia. We would test our theories about how the world worked with travel and observation in distant lands. We had already made the decision not to live in Australia. Learning about the land and indigenous people took over three years of part-time travel. We would spend three to five months each year traveling and camping in the Outback; learning about plants, animals, and the ancient ways of the aboriginal people.

Gain More Wisdom from Those Who Came Before You

The oldest known tribe on the planet is the indigenous people of Australia. While some controversy exists over the exact time frame, it is probably close to 40,000 years that the Aborigines have existed in uninterrupted society. Think about that compared to the Anglo European or American Indian. It is literally 10 times the history of any other people on the planet. Despite this feat, they are some of the worst treated and almost eradicated species on Earth.

To us, it was as if Australia was a large loaf of bread and we could tear off small bits and feed ourselves for a very long time. The loaf never seemed to end and it tasted good.

Again, with a theme of mortality, I looked at this society with perplexed admiration. How did they do it? What philosophy allowed them to span a legacy for so many thousands of years in harmony with the environment? This was a riddle worth looking into. It appeared that the disease culture of the pure native did not exist. Everything was in perfect harmony in the Aboriginal world. The harsh environment was a candy store of richness and history if you knew how to use it. How did they do it?

Diet Could Be Key

Referring back to my farming experience, I examined the varied diet of the Aboriginal. Some estimates counted over 300 types of food in their diet. The sad thing is that when you confine these people to a Westernized diet, they cannot thrive any longer. In fact, their ability to metabolize refined carbohydrates is very limited and alcohol, the – super sugar – is an addictive poison to their systems.

Political Struggles Always Play a Role

Huge social and political problems face Australia. Yet, aside from all the strife and hardship endured since the arrival of the "white fella," their true spirit still shines through.

The separation of the world into compartments is a mental construct of the Cartesian system of logic. It was never considered an option to ancient Aboriginals. In fact, the cosmos and planet were connected without question. Everything in the world had spiritual significance at the deepest level, and this was held in memory to be celebrated with song at any instance. This was a completely different society. Isolated from the rest of the world, the Aboriginals developed in isolation over the course of 40,000 years. The average person in ancient Australia lived and died in a tribe that had a migratory existence.

This held great interest for me, as I too had been migrating all over the planet. What could these mysterious people teach me about living longer and better? It had worked perfectly until the Europeans arrived. The consequent conflict is one of the worst examples of social and human injustice the human race has ever created. I suggest that it is 200 years of genocide, coarse and underpinned by the British colonists. Not being British or a bigot, I was able to witness the beauty and plight of these Aboriginal peoples.

After three and a half years of study, I came to the conclusion that this unique and isolated tribe of almost a million people in 1788 was and is one of the most advanced species on the planet. As a people, they have developed right-brain dominance, rich with special verbal, musical, and visual capacity. Their story is more advanced than any other race of people I have ever encountered. We, as a counter-point race, cannot even communicate with the Aboriginal well enough to be able to measure their intelligence. Yet, as little as 50 years ago scientists and society have judged them as a subspecies.

This ignorance and arrogance continues in Australia today. The country is rife with indigenous turmoil and many unanswered questions about how to create a lasting Aboriginal lifestyle in a modern world. The struggle is, in fact, similar to the problem we all face today. Our planet is going to cull the weak ones, and the shocking news is that eight out of ten are the weak ones! Do we want to pay this price with our children's blood? I think not when we look at it this way. However, the Australian Aboriginal is truly a mirror of our planetary problems, only on a smaller scale.

The Message is the Same Regardless of the Culture

Diversity of diet, spiritual harmony, and unending awareness were the same messages I learned in Chinese medicine and here they were again in this indigenous tribe. I was beginning to see a pattern. Perhaps, I could live another full six months? My spirit was soaring with the newly appreciated knowledge and I layered it atop investigations into pre-Buddhist Vedic history. This was completing the loop of understanding in Chinese medicine and Taoist philosophy. Ayurveda as a system of healthcare is the oldest written form of medicine on the planet. It is over 5000 years old and is responsible for the development of Chinese medicine.

Ayurveda came from the three-element system or Tri-Dosha of fire, water, and air. Taking these three elements, the Chinese system added two others – wood and metal. All systems of health use the elements of fire, water and air to summarize, in relatable terms, the living and functional world around them. As I continued to study physiology, biochemistry, and nutrition, it struck me how the philosophical systems of the ancient ones could actually be used in modern science without too much conflict. In fact, parallels had already been published between ancient Vedic teachings about the cosmos and current theory at the University of California Berkeley.

This was quantum physics and the work of Fritjof Capra, Ph.D. that were included in his book, *The Tao of Physics.*

I was developing a holistic view of the universe and a way that I could actually continue to live in it. The ancient sciences were as valid as quantum physics in my fight to stay on the planet. The internal dialog of just how to do life with certainty every day was in fact just that: a dialog, which aided the observation of daily events and served as a guide to navigation through the massive amounts of information I was trying to process.

In one sense, I was like Homer's Ulysses, looking for my beloved homeland. Held somewhere between my head and my heart, a peace must be found in this lifetime. The circle of life had become full and complete, and as the years of self-imposed study drifted in Nelson, I was roused with an uneasy feeling that a bigger picture existed. There had to be a unifying theory, one that put to rest any question of doubt. This theory must include science and heartfelt faith of a righteous path that was superior to what was previously available. Was I asking too much? I did not feel I was. In fact, I felt the answers were very close, and that the "dust of illusion was waiting to be removed from my eyes."

I went looking for the Holy Grail, both inwardly and outwardly, and this is disruptive to any relationship. I was swimming towards an unknown distant shore, knowing it was a desperate life-challenging event. Doing this left no security for M. I quickly learned that I could not return to the raft, I had pursued a path of following truth and had allowed the universe to lead me. I had to remain open and vigilant to my quest. It was a life lived consciously, healthfully, and with purpose!

The inner quest had ramifications on my relationship, ones I never saw coming. M had been there with me and for me during medical school, after graduating, in practice, through my cancer, and during my retirement. But it was my restlessness and internally focused struggle that ended my relationship with M in 1995. We had been in each other's company every day for 18 years. The raft of attachment was breaking up in the sea of life, and this was disconcerting and painful, but all the study about the Tao was helping me cope.

As one pushes the mental and emotional boundaries of daily existence, you must be willing to accept change at all levels. M and I were inseparable, however, over the next five years that relationship would have to be sacrificed for the sake of further personal development.

Whatever it took, life had to be lived, and sometimes the mental constraints of relationships get in the way. Rinpoche reflected once on this; he thought that those who entered relationships were "very brave," as he could not have the courage to take responsibility for another in that way... "Very difficult," he would say. Being independent in thought and not relying on another was a hurdle that had to be jumped if full realization was to be achieved.

Right or wrong at the time, ending the relationship seemed to be a positive move for both of us. Gratefully, we are still friends and confidants on our journeys. We both have new partners and we occasionally visit each other's home with support and reverence for our history shared. She leads a gentle life in the US and New Zealand, floating between the two. Life is perfect if you let it be.

A Higher Purpose and Vow Always Should Be Considered Important

Does one always know there is a higher purpose to their life? I think so. The feelings of insignificance of one's life can vanish, seeing the complete trust placed in a parent by a baby's gaze. The connection is that simple. Trust, love, and commitment are the invisible adhesives, holding life together so it can be stitched into solid fabric.

This fabric gives shape and texture to a life, short or long; it's your life and you have to wear your fabric every day. What had I just been given? Wow! I was still alive and had learned so little about so much. How could I ever hope to find the unifying theory of life?

Khensur Thabkhey Rinpoche, a Tibetan Lama mentioned previously, was 800 years old when I first met him. This man had chosen over and over, for the last eight centuries to be reincarnated to the same purpose – to teach with compassion, His Holiness, the Dalai Lama. Rinpoche was from a long line of Lamas dedicated to being personal tutors to the Dalai Lama; each time he was reincarnated to his path. It's not just H.H. that comes back each lifetime to teach; there is a whole support team. In the later years of his physical existence, he was sent to New Zealand to expound the Dharma to those who would listen. This was not the first Lama I had met, but he was the Lama for me. He and I had an understanding early in our meeting. I had work to do and what he held in his head was integral to my work. I took my vows with him and never looked back; I knew it was the right path.

The Bodhisattva Vow expounds that one must do all that is necessary to achieve a life with high merit and mastery. Respectful and dutiful to all the common responsibilities, one is asked to reach for enlightenment in this life and then when one is able to leap into unending bliss, come back and join the masses until all reach the same equanimitable space. This was what I was meant to do and I sensed it. My pain and brush with death had been a preparation for a knowledge that could reduce or eliminate the pain in others. When practised, this unifying code of conduct would allow those who wanted liberation to achieve it, but I was not Buddha! What was I going to teach?

Khensur Thabkhey Rinpoche had a method, and as I absorbed all that my turtle-egg-thick skull could, the genius of this man burst forth from my heart. My lesson had been easy for the Lama to see, once examined from an unattached and enlightened point of view. Overcome all adversity, go to school, become a doctor, overcome terminal cancer, educate yourself to a higher level, and spend your life teaching the methods of health, discovered and refined over a lifetime.

Rinpoche pointed out how "STARK" the message was! He thought it was hilarious, too. That was it! It was the birth of STARK HEALTH as a concept of simplicity and clarity.

Dharma is so simple. I was even given the name of my method with my birth; but there was still much work ahead. To write the unifying code of the Universe in just a few pages was easy, Einstein had done it! What I needed was another language if anyone else was expected to read it. I left New Zealand and returned to the US to allow passion and vision to unite. What actually happened was a lot different than I expected, but exactly what you would expect according to Rinpoche. It would take another 10 years to bring the concept to fullness.

Why Not Help Others with What I Knew?

I had an idea. I could write my newly formed idea and distribute it via this newly developing technology called the Internet. It was 1997, and I was living on an "island" outside Nelson at the end of a very long farm road. I went online! Progress was very slow, but bit-by-bit, I began to compile the information for the website – whatever that was. At around 1100 pages on the computer, it was time to take a breather. Mom's health was failing, so I decided to skip the New Zealand winter and go to the United States.

Riding the Air Waves Was Similar to Riding the Waves in Life

During 1996, I had discovered a new sport, one that filled me with passion and adventure. It was paragliding! As described by another flier from Scotland, "You take a bag of laundry, walk to the top of a perfectly good hill, inflate it and jump off into thin air." Paragliding was the three dimensional surfing I had been looking for. Concerned about the amount of time it was taking out of my life, Rinpoche encouraged me to investigate "passion" and saw it as a good thing.

The previous winter I had been to Europe and had competed in a dozen or so international competitions. Paragliding is similar to yacht racing. Landmarks are used as buoys, with the fastest one around the course winning. The courses vary from 20 to 60 miles depending on the weather, and are designed to drop about 90 percent of the field along the way to the goal. Walking with a 20-kilogram pack on your back, hitchhiking through the countryside, just adds to the mystique of this sport.

I packed the paraglider and headed for California. My mission, secondary to my mother's health, was to represent New Zealand in an international competition in Aspen. Little did I know how it was soon to change my life.

The problem with Aspen is that those who are rich consume unending amounts of resources. I could not believe that a campground with a shower in it could not be found in a 50-mile radius when there were so many mansions on the hillside! After a cold night sleeping in my car in the canyon at a place aptly named "Difficult," (to an enlightened one, this should have been a clue!) I went to town the next morning for a cup of hot coffee. Sunny and warm, I sat and just soaked up the mountain air. The next thing I knew, a very attractive lady, with an equally handsome boxer dog, asked if they could join my table. "No worries, mate," I said. The future Mrs. Stark sat down and a conversation began.

An Achievement Worth a Pat on the Back

I managed to finish amongst the top dozen US pilots at the competition and stayed in Aspen for the season, smitten with my new friend. As I was going back to New Zealand in the southern spring, I made plans to leave. Sharon and I were getting serious; it seemed like we were a great match. She was a medical doctor with a specialty in radiology; I was a chiropractor with an interest in all things including high-level training in radiology, so I could at least understand her language. She was outgoing, athletic, and had a lifestyle of her own making.

By fate or destiny, I'm not sure which, I asked her to marry me prior to boarding the plane for my return to New Zealand. I was to return within a month, with glider and possessions in hand, momentarily turning my back on New Zealand.

If one has to live in the United States, Aspen is about as good as it gets. A town of about 5000, it boasts Gucci, Lauren, Prada, and Fendi outlets just to make a statement to the world. This, combined with the beautiful mountains and cooler summers, make it a haven, sought after by the rich and often not-so-famous. With my work from the last eight-to-ten years on hold, I amused myself, how enamored I was with it all. As the winter set in, I realized I was about to learn to ski for the first time. How much fun could one have!

Developing the website to which Rinpoche had given me the name, "StarkHealth," was a project worth the work. Also, slipping on the boots, walking to the Gondola every day and soaking in the steam room in the afternoon at "The Aspen Club" has to be as good as it gets in the USA. I skied over 100 days that winter, adding another sport to my belt. Was I losing my way, my spiritual path in the land of the rich and famous? New Zealand called. By the following year, Sharon and I were on our way back to Christchurch.

How my life and focus had changed in this time! We lived in the city and began our new life – but it didn't work. By the following year we had moved back to Aspen, restless with both the changing world and ourselves. The Universe would have lessons to teach me whether I was interested or not. Letting go is something not all people can do. You have to negotiate your boundaries when you become at one with your own death, not everyone can do that, and as the relationship with Sharon went on, it became clear over the years that defining my own boundaries would be a lesson learned.

The Invisible Magnetism in Life

Magnetism is one of the first experiments I recall from school science projects. Iron filings are placed on a piece of paper and a magnet is pulled underneath the paper to move the iron filings "invisibly." With this simple experiment, one can see that which is unseeable: the effect of magnetism. Aspen was similar. While we had ideological problems with it, we were pulled back. It was just like a magnet.

In the summer of 1999, we attended a weeklong medical conference in Snowmass, Colorado, on Wilderness Medicine. At the seminar was Dr. Ron Rothenburg, M.D. who talked about Anti-Aging Medicine. He claimed that the hormonal system was the master link to the aging process, and everything else depended on it, including pathology. I paid attention; this was the first time I had ever heard a medical doctor make sense about the topic of health, prevention and a rationale for reversing physical decline.

Sharon was off to California and immediately signed up with Rothenburg as a patient. I observed the process and was intrigued by the tenets, but not the practice. While I could see the science behind the decline of hormones and how they opened the door for accelerated aging processes, I disagreed with the idea that prescription hormones were a quick fix to put life in order. Anti-aging medicine tenets state that the hormone level of a healthy, active 25-to-35-year-old is what exceptionally fit and healthy people have, regardless of age. If we mimic these levels in a 50-, 60-, or 70-year-old with prescription medications, they should feel like their younger counterpart. And they did.

I decided to study the topic more in-depth, and attended my first Anti-Aging Medicine Conference in Chicago. I could feel the energy in that room of 5000 doctors. For the first time, interventional medicine could actually work preventively. As a chiropractor, I had always embraced the ideal of preventative care. Patients would come monthly for "tune-ups" to stimulate their nervous system via manipulation and thus modulate their organ and muscular system to function better – before illness occurred. For close to 100 years, this has been the chiropractic way. Now the very same people who called us quacks discovered it was true all along. Prevention is the cure, Lifestyle is the Medicine!

I realized that the rest of the world was slowly waking up to my new field of endeavor. The hormone theory of aging had merit, and the effects of lifestyle on health were actually greater than any drug in the majority of cases. In fact, Allen Mintz, M.D., the founder of Cenegenics, a very successful Age Management Clinic in Las Vegas, reported "Over 90 percent of patients could achieve optimal hormone levels with just the judicious use of lifestyle." This confirmed everything I had learned from the Vedic, Chinese, chiropractic, and medical fields; but how could I put it in a capsule and sell it to the world? I mean, it involved sweat and effort, two additives people don't like!

Over the next few years I would move back to New Zealand three more times. Moving can be a distinct stressor in life. Because I had done it so many times in my life, I had learned to detach from the stress of moving and uprooting one's life. However, I believe it was more difficult for Sharon to move and the stresses caught up with her. It was an intense moment in my life, as the emotional liability of my relationship and its effects on my health were seen for the first time. I had let myself slide physically for the first time since my recovery from chemo. It was not Sharon's fault; it was my lesson if I chose to learn it. I vowed to regain my strength, composition, and focus. I had learned to set boundaries of what was, and was not in my personal environment and relationships. A painful, poignant lesson learned and we began the "divorce process" in 2006.

Couldn't Resist the Urge to Help Others Heal

Anti-aging medicine appeared to be such a major part of the puzzle of human health. I dreamed about the potential of this new body of knowledge to help patients. It wasn't long before I was convinced that anti-aging medicine worked. I began seeing patients in my clinic in Christchurch in 2007. By 2008, I had a personal assistant and actual objective proof that my patient population was doing as well or better than those on hormone replacement therapy. I had arrived, and the information was slotting into place at a very fast pace. A rationale now existed for a natural, non-pharmaceutical anti-aging practice based on lifestyle, which could be objectively proven.

My patients had proven to me, as I had proved to myself, that the body could function better with less risk, and possibly longer. It was a guarantee for quality of life for anyone who was willing to follow the program. While I practised what I preached to my patients, the two-and-a-half days of patient contact time was becoming an increasingly busy schedule. I needed to perfect a method of education for my patients as well as a method of teaching other doctors the high standards required to do this work. Again, the Universe supplied the answer in the form of a charismatic Australian teacher named Matt Church, a self-made guru of the media arts, writer, speaker, mentor, coach, and the like. I quickly learned better methods of communication and embraced many of his ideas as superior methods of facilitation for patients and doctors. I was back in the fast lane this time, but it had taken 20 additional years of training to realize just how precious the mission was. As Matt would tell me, "Patterson, you have to accept that you are the Guru of Anti-Aging and Lifestyle Medicine, and teach with passion and conviction."

Reflections on the Journey

The journey from sitting on my sofa, crying softly to myself with the acceptance of my death just 20 years prior, to having in my hands today, the most advanced system of personal mental and physical health is astounding. I remain humbled by the blessing and opportunity at hand. I am humbled by the fact that people I do not know will read these words and take meaning from them, and then return to their families to take actions that will improve the quality of their daily life. I am humbled by the fact this information and these simple actions compound, like interest, and it's daily interest! Any banker will agree that's the best kind.

In addition to the physical blessings, I have to acknowledge that as a man and individual in a modern time, I have not been an easy person to live with or be around. We all must take responsibility for our own actions and what we will allow to happen in our interpersonal relationships. For many years, I was unclear of what role I wanted to play or was expected to play in the game of life with my partner. Now, when the pain of divorce made me get clear about what were the most important things to have, an incredible thing happened – an angel appeared!

In one way I defined my perfect partner via the positive and negative experiences I had in the past and what I "thought" I would want going forward. Who showed up was an amazing person, one who had also been on her personal development path for the last 20 years. She had done the work and understood what I had discovered about personal growth – it's never really done. The joy of being where you are, the joy of being with whom you're with, at the time you are there, has defined a peacefulness and intensity to "now" that was unknown to me previously. Gayel in every way has allowed this process of passion in life to continue with physical and spiritual support. The days that are numbered and yet to be counted are insignificant, as all are a gift.

With gratitude, I awaken each day with two questions on my mind. 1) Am I breathing? If I am, then it's a great day and 2) How are you, Patterson, going to give something back to this planet today? With self-love and gratitude, I can do anything! The passion of answering the question makes me hop out of bed and get started!

Well, everything is connected to everything. I need to have a strong body, nourished by the best food available, and lastly I need a dash of passion about my goals this day. Planning for success, I know when to work out, what to eat, and when to take private time. With what some would consider exceptionally low goals for the day, I now have a platform for success.

Decisions to Live Affect More Than Just Ourselves

In medical school, one of the first courses we take is Gross Anatomy. We identify the landmarks on the surface that orient us to the structures that are below. We go deeper into the subject and take a course in Surgical Anatomy, not missing a stitch of tissue along the way. I remember my examination one day with a pin in the abdomen of the cadaver and the question: From the surface to the deepest structure, name each layer of tissue.

This is similar to what happens in life. As you look at the world you live in and make decisions for yourself and your loved ones, you affect them and yourself both on the surface and to the deepest parts of their being. All this happens with simple decisions on how to live each day.

I remember the feeling of being overwhelmed when I started med school. You, dear reader, may be overwhelmed with the health issues that arise in your life. However, once you learn to manipulate your environment to your advantage, this sense will disappear. You need to know two things: Firstly, what is the gross anatomy of the situation – where all this started and all the death traps and disease risks you are taking with your life? And secondly, what is the surgical anatomy of the situation – how do you live with gratitude, humility, and a sense of purpose? I call this amazing process "STARK HEALTH," the direct uncluttered view of the structure and function of health. With these tools, you can protect that which is so very precious... life. It is not a guarantee; just a higher probability of a successful outcome.

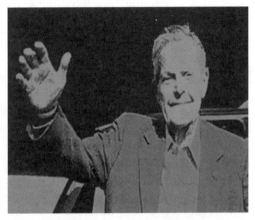

Dr. George Goodheart, D.C. (1918 – 2008)

A few days before his passing waving farewell to his students; an example of a brilliant life, lived with passion and dignity. He has inspired me to continue a lifelong ambition to learn, share and stay positive - to be what you want to see in the world – Thank you George!

LIVE NOW – DIE LATER

PART TWO

Your world – where your risk comes from – is hidden from your view

CHAPTER EIGHT
The Landscape of Life – Your Life

How would you plan your funeral? At the age of 34, planning mine was no picnic. In my head, sitting in my quiet condo overlooking eight lanes of the San Diego freeway, it was easy to understand I was a doctor, jaded by personal experience, and overwhelmed with technical knowledge. I could not focus on my funeral. I wanted to live; however, I had a very real timeline of immediacy and I was floundering. What would be the most effective method of investigation and more importantly, what would yield the ultimate result of staying above ground? I had to not only "cheat death," I had to master life! It was obvious I had not gotten this right – so far.

Practicality and immediacy were my partners. Research was a luxury. Application of life-saving skills was a priority. A decision had to be made about how to outlive the projections of imminent death. I decided to split my agenda, starting with what I knew instinctively – going to the ancient ones for practical knowledge about how to eat, sleep, and keep breathing. The second part was to return to science for useful application. This part was what I knew best.

The physical body has needs: food, air, water, rest, and touch, and connection to other living beings. As elemental as it sounds, this is what sustains life. At this point in my life, I could not afford to miss anything on my list of needs. I had to muster all elements to be of the highest quality.

What Can I Eliminate From My Life When Every Moment Counts?

When negative thoughts came up, I let them go, I had no time for them. When hunger set in, only the highest quality food would do. I knew it was important not to get locked into a fanatical crusade of any diet.

Nutritional supplements were formulated and used three times per day. Lastly, I ran farther each day. I felt better. I asked better questions of myself, such as, what I expected to learn about the tragedy that had been my life before the cancer?

Where did life go so horribly wrong? Was I a victim of chance, a random lottery of life, someone that had been in the wrong place at the wrong time? Could I influence this process at all? Every cell in my body told me this new reality could be. Finding out how to manifest a new reality was the question. It began with the mind itself. As I had been taught from day one in med school, "Healing manifests from the top down and the inside out." I had to start at the top!!

Where do thoughts come from and what is my reality? The trillions of cells in the body are physically made of molecules supplied by the food you eat, the air you breathe, the thoughts you have and the water you drink. But where do thoughts actually come from? Who was responsible for putting the molecules together which made up the physical body? What was the grand design? My Lama said, "It was beyond us mortals to know what was the intention of who helped nurture life in the first place because we were only human and could not comprehend it." But with little time left to live, these were the real questions I asked myself just after my return from the North Shore of Oahu during the week I finished chemotherapy.

To continue living, I needed to use the tools I had at my disposal. It was clear in my mind that I needed to return to what I knew as a scientist. I also had to ask basic questions to understand how to avoid future conflicts emotionally that may have negative effects on my health. What would it be like after chemotherapy with an immune system that didn't work? You don't want to get a cold; it could kill you! How and where do you begin? There aren't any drugs that will make any difference at all. There is not one proven method that works better than others at reducing your risk of catching a cold. Do you have any power over the process? With all of these questions in my head, I remembered a good book I had read in medical school about the origin of modern health decline. I would start there.

The Urgency of Astounding Facts about Nutrition and Physical Degeneration

Weston A. Price was a dentist who had asked similar questions in the beginning of the 20th century. He wasn't sick at the time though. He was an exceptional dentist that had observed a decline in the dental health of his patients over the course of his professional career. Once retired, he looked for answers to the questions and how best to find those answers.

As a lucky break, Price's brother-in-law worked for National Geographic Magazine. Price poured time into looking at the pictures from distant lands and was impressed by primitive tribes' people with beautiful, healthy-looking smiles. Was there a relationship between diet and dental health? He realized he did not know what "normal" people looked like. As any scientist would, he needed to collect data, so he set about traveling the world to ask this primary question: Does the modern diet have any effect on dental health and overall health?

Price had to examine and accurately record the diet and dental health of "primitive" civilizations. In addition, if he found populations that had switched to a Western diet, he could compare dental and general health issues in that population. Price traveled to find these secluded pockets of humanity, ones that were untouched by Western civilization. It took close to a decade of painstaking work to publish the compendium of knowledge he gathered from his travels. His work is respected and revered the world over as the authoritative classic on nutrition; it chronicles the effects of modern foods as the cause of decline for our species.

In the foreword to the epic publication *Nutrition and Physical Degeneration*, Earnest A. Hooton of Harvard University wrote:

> Since we have known for a long time that savages have excellent teeth and that civilized men have terrible teeth, it seems to me that we have been extraordinarily stupid in concentrating all of our attention upon the task of finding out why teeth are so poor without ever bothering to learn why savage teeth are good? Dr. Weston Price seems to be the only person with the scientific horse sense to supplement his knowledge of the probable causes of dental disease with the study of the dietary regimens, which are associated with dental health.

The year was 1938.

It had taken him over 10 years of traveling the world to accumulate the authoritative data that was necessary to draw the conclusion about what health requirements were necessary to promote not only healthy teeth, but also the health of people. And back then, he didn't have airplanes to take him to these hidden populations.

The results of his research started the field of therapeutic nutrition and influenced some of the earliest research on the existence of vitamins and minerals. How fortunate I had been to be exposed to this work in my early days of medical school. Sure, I had very much ignored the depth of the work, coming away with a simple conclusion – eat better and live longer. However, the solution was much deeper than that. The very subtle implications were only obvious upon closer inspection of the work. They impacted me so much in my life I feel compelled to share them with you, as they will show you how and why food is critical.

Diverging for just a moment, I could have written a book just about my philosophy about health and what I learned through my entire cancer episode in life, but how effective would that have been? Here I have a chance to expose you to the same original research that I read years ago that changed my life. If it was powerful enough to change my life, it could also change yours. Price's work gave me the strong foundation that I needed as a reason to modify my life. Standalone facts and physiology rarely do that.

So, dear reader, use the resources provided to look at The Weston A. Price Foundation and the supportive work of his contemporary Sally Fallon and make this your discovery process as well.

After reading Price's work again, I realized that I had to repair the weak link in the chain of my life and my DNA. The topography of the living landscape is where we get our landmarks from to keep our bearings. Well, I didn't feel I had a clue as to which direction I was going in at that time, but Price answered the question with a scientific eloquence that was distinguished and timely. The fact is that it had been sitting on the shelf for 50 years was of no relevance to me.

The most understated fact of all that I have learned is so simple and horrific: Diet changes life. Dr. Weston A. Price's work can never be repeated, as we no longer have pure civilizations to compare against modern diets. Coca Cola has made it to every corner of the globe, often before the explorers themselves. But the facts are there and they are tied to the history of each and every one of us.

CHAPTER NINE

Anatomy of a Dream – What Healthy People Do

As a chiropractor, I knew about bone health. But here was Dr. Price, a dentist who was teaching me how bone health and the health of teeth were keys to the immune system and structural integrity of the body. These "keys" were essential if I wanted to have some certainty about how to stay above ground, given my current history.

We Deform Our Skeletons by Eating Processed Foods

As we eat more processed and de-mineralized foods, we can see the structures of our loved ones actually deforming their skeletons. Yes, you read that sentence correctly; we can see the deformation of the skeleton in our loved ones. And you can see the deformation in those you don't know well, too. If our body is young and growing, the facial bones cannot achieve the maximum growth when a processed diet is eaten. Price documented a direct correlation between crowded teeth in the upper and lower jaw and the amount of processed food a person ate during developmental childhood (below the age of 25). He recorded decreased resistance to illness and loss of physical stature in those on processed food diets. Look around you and see who has crowded teeth in the upper and/or lower jaw. Ask them questions about their diet, their parents' diet and their grandparents' diet.

Moody? Cry a Lot? Depressed? It's Your Diet You Must Change

What was even more astounding were the effects observed on a society's mental health. In the primitive or untouched societies, he observed a happy, cheerful population where good humor was abundant and curiosity endemic. In addition, wherever Price was, he was awestruck by the fact that he rarely heard a crying baby. *Children were happy, inquisitive, and calm.* Do we really need three out of ten children on medication for sadness, dullness, and bursts of frustration? I think not. We need to medicate our thinking with common sense... and a good diet.

Look around you and see how many people have happy babies that don't cry. How many have children that aren't on medications? Check to see how many of your friends are happy and not on medications themselves.

Dr. Price made a major discovery, but in the early part of the last century, the comparisons of modern living with this utopian existence were met with disbelief. While Dr. Price's work was of the highest scientific standard of the day, it had one major flaw. In his conclusion, he asked people to take responsibility for themselves by eating a wholesome diet and being physically active. This was the antithesis of what modern life was attesting at the time. Progress was inevitable and it was science and technology that would make the world a better, easier more convenient place to live. Science and technology were the saviors. The perturbations of human biology were clearly visible.

Modern Day Life Must Be Considered

Price's research was almost heresy in light of the day it was published. How backwards a conclusion he had proposed. Perhaps it was valid but not practical! Surely science would find the answers to these questions if it tried? Big Pharmacy was just beginning to get a firm foothold, as was larger scale agriculture. The farm and cityscapes were changing in the modern world. The supply of basic foodstuffs and their milling practices had changed remarkably inside of 30 years. Our basic diet had made its first real shift in human history when we introduced refined foods to our diet. As a result we were paying a high price in terms of our health. My quest seemed to have found a basic truth. It is important to restate in Price's words what he had learned from the "savages" for whom he had the utmost respect:

"Life in all its fullness is Mother Nature obeyed." –W. A. Price

The truly healthy people of the planet were not the ones with the most possessions or sophisticated scientific technology. Instead, they were the ones that obeyed the laws of Mother Nature. It was the last few untouched, primitive societies that taught Dr. Price the code of healthy living.

The Diet-Health Connection is Real

Healthy food is fundamental to a healthy life. The basic considerations need to be examined if one is to understand what and how our own diseases begin. Cancer, diabetes, heart disease, premature dementia, autoimmune dysfunction, osteoporosis, and stroke are all symptoms of massive malnutrition, malformation, or both. We have inherited an unsafe world and are passing genocide onto our children. Just last night on the evening news, a researcher, Dr. Peter Gluckman, reported that obesity was genetic!

> Scientists from the Liggins Institute in New Zealand, say it is possible we have a genetic switch

putting us down a thin or fat pathway from birth and there's not a lot we can do about it. The reason 50 percent of the population is now obese is due to prenatal gene regulation. The only hope of influence over the genes is proper nutrition for the mother from pre-conception and throughout the pregnancy.

-Gluckman
(Dr. Price's observation – 50 years previously)

And that's not all. It's startling that over one-third of women have improper prenatal nutrition in this day and age. If one-third of women have improper prenatal nutrition and this influences the developing fetus, causing obesity, most of us are doomed to a life of poor health. Had Price still been alive to hear this report he would have been displeased and possibly frustrated that no one had heeded his message. The tenets of his research are as pointed today as they were to me 30 years ago. They warrant repeating.

What We Can Do to Reverse Our Negative Genetic Codes

Since we cannot turn back the clock and have the luxury of a cleaner, better environment, people need to have a basic understanding of environments necessary for a long and healthy life. With the amount of apparent pain in society, I hope we will find a more receptive audience for this empowering message. In 30 years of earnest investigation, the following is the most inconvenient truth about the human condition. The prescription is painless.

The prescription for a genetically supported human race:

1. Reduce the volume of industrial effluents, including fluorides, now contaminating our air, water and food, as rapidly as possible, through federal, state, and local controls.

2. Ban the use of untested food additives immediately. Reduce the number of those tested, considered harmless and approved for their use, to an absolute minimum.

3. Rapidly phase out the use of long-acting pesticides and herbicides unless proven harmless, or in emergency situations such as malaria control. Ban the sale of these pesticides for household use. Seek control of insect pests through other means, including soil improvement. Well-nourished plants are more resistant to insects and fungi than deficient ones.

4. Warn the public that all petrochemicals, whether in food, water, air pesticides, cosmetics, detergents, drugs, or other environmental contacts, are potentially dangerous to many and probably all individuals. Tell them minimal contact is the best.

5. Give the public access to fundamental knowledge of good nutrition. (Especially children) If we are to survive, this must be taught in every school grade from kindergarten through college. Primitive wisdom tells us that the production of healthy, normal babies depends upon optimum prenatal nutrition *both prior to conception and during pregnancy.* Breastfeeding is most important and should be followed by a diet high in raw and unprocessed foods.

Most birth deformities are unnecessary reflections of environmental circumstances prior to birth and prior to conception.

6. Good bones, good muscles, attractive skin, normal endocrines, a healthy liver, good reproductive capacity, good food values, and nourishing food are not necessarily expensive. Even now, many Russian peasants subsist primarily on vegetable soup, hard rye bread, and occasional bits of meat. Their teeth and health are reported to be superior.

7. Compost city wastes for use as fertilizers. Return organic materials, minerals and trace elements to help rebuild our plundered soil and reduce the use of synthetic fertilizers high in nitrogen content which are contaminating our water and food supplies. Demonstrate to farmers that this approach is economically feasible.

8. Grow foods for quality rather that quantity. High-vitamin and high-mineral foods have much higher nutritional value that those with more calories but fewer essential nutrients. Calories alone are not enough.

9. In line with the concepts of biochemical individuality, as expressed by Dr. Rodger Williams who postulates the inheritance of acquired partial enzyme blocks, many patients need vitamin and mineral supplements for optimal health and even for normal metabolism. These must be prescribed, along with a basic diet, as deemed necessary by the experience and knowledge of the individual practitioner.

10. Aside from a study of nutritional values of food, which most people will not undertake, there are a few simple steps available to everyone. If these steps were to be

publicized and universally followed, the immediate and long-term benefits would be incalculable and the results would certainly be obvious in six months.

They are as follows:

a. Reduce the consumption of sugar in all forms to an absolute minimum.

b. WHITE OUT! Avoid white and ordinary whole wheat bread. Eat only whole grain breads made from freshly ground flour, free of chemical preservatives. (The production of such bread would require a mill and adequate bakeries in every community). Use brown in place of white polished rice. These simple changes in food production and habits would result in a much higher intake of protein, Vitamin B complex, minerals, and Vitamin E. The latter has only recently been recognized as essential for man. (It is appalling to think of the millions of tons of these vital nutrients that have been extracted from our foods and fed to animals over the past century.) Since this time we have learned the hybrid wheat of today is a major contributor to bad health, so no wheat, rye, or barley.

c. When available, use only fresh fruits, vegetables, dark green leaves of lettuce, and other greens such as watercress that have been raised in fertile soil without the use of insecticides. Ordinary fruits should be peeled because of possible pesticide residues and vegetables thoroughly washed for the same reason. Home gardens are to be encouraged. Frozen or canned vegetables and fruits are nourishing, but less desirable. Steam or lightly cook all vegetables that are not eaten raw. Save any cooking water for tomato juice cocktails or soup.

d. Sprouted beans, alfalfa, and other seeds contain desirable nutrients and are free of contamination. They can be sprouted in every kitchen. The consumption of 60 percent or more of food in the uncooked state is desirable.

e. Avoid stale fats and foods cooked in recycled fats, such as ordinary potato chips, French fried potatoes, etc. Recent preliminary evidence advanced by Robert S. Ford suggests that rancid fats, rather than animal fats per se, may be one of the real villains responsible for atherosclerosis. Sources of stale fat include products such as bread, crackers, pastries, and commercial cereals made from stored flour. (This is talking about trans fatty acids over 50 years ago.)

f. Two serving daily of foods with an alkaline residue such as potatoes, unsprayed beet greens, turnip tops, spinach, dandelion greens, dehydrated grasses, or sorghum cane juices, in accordance with the findings of Dr. Martha R. Jones, may be of great importance in maintaining the body's alkali reserves. Her studies suggest that good diets providing a moderate excess of alkali to neutralize acid foods such as meat, bread, eggs and other nutritious staples are not only beneficial to health, but are major factors in the prevention of dental caries. This is one of the few aspects of native diets not analyzed by Dr. Price.

The comments made as a summary of Price's work by Granville F. Knight over 50 years ago still ring true today. Applying these tenets can have the same impact on your health that they have had on mine. That's why I am so excited to share them with you. The benefits you get will include superior health, reduced risk of degenerative disease and perhaps, straight teeth in your kids! As I discovered, fame and fortune are of little reward when the Grim Reaper is knocking at your door.

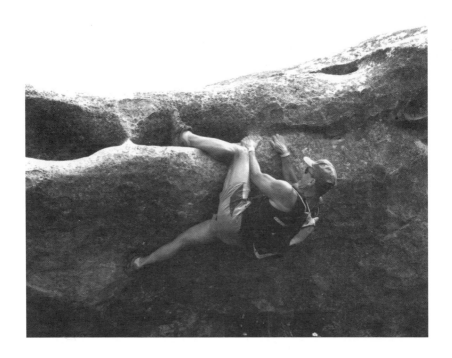

Life is the challenge. Metaphors are the actions we take to actually convince ourselves we are fully alive. Find your rock and start climbing! I am only 3 feet off the ground in the photo above – but at 63 I am committed. Good food, family, friends and time to work with yourself. Precious!

CHAPTER TEN

Nutrition and Physical Degeneration
The Scientific Experiment That Can
Never Be Repeated

In China, the Taoist's talk of The Way is specifically referring to the Way of Life, a life that is rich, colorful, and immune to the ravages of time. The "Living Immortals" were physical testaments that the tenets actually worked. The Adepts who devoted their lives to the practices and formulae set down by centuries of scholarly research were rewarded with a lifespan and legendary health span well into their hundreds.

Imagine being a capable martial artist at the age of 110! Legend or fact, when I read the formula of The Way, the scientist in me said, this is very plausible. For someone who was in my predicament, I followed and gained benefits out of the ordinary, which yielded the miraculous!

Where's the Proof?

I wanted proof in my modern world about the quintessential habits that locked in immunity, vitality, strength, and spirit. You probably want more proof as well.

A closer inspection of Dr. Price's work confirmed early premonitions. As Price said, "Instead of the customary procedure of analyzing the expression of degeneration as modern scientific research does, *a search has been made for groups to be used as controls who are largely free from these afflictions.*"

It was as simple as that. In every instance, he located groups of primitive peoples that were immune to the diseases of the modern world. His quest was to isolate the common traits and subject them to further scientific tests.

Considering the travel methods and distances covered in the late 1920s and early 1930s, the completeness of his work is astounding. Isolated and modernized groups were studied in the following areas:

- Switzerland
- the Gaelics in Outer and Inner Hebrides
- the Eskimos of Alaska
- the Indians in the far North, West, and Central Canada, Western United States, and Florida
- the Melanesians and Polynesians of eight archipelagoes in the Southern Pacific
- tribes in Eastern and Central Africa
- the Aborigines of Australia
- the Maori of New Zealand
- the ancient civilizations and their descendants in Peru both along the coast, in the Sierras, and in the Amazon basin

Dr. Price also studied the modernized white populations in these areas, when available, as a comparison.

Dr. Price's Discovery Still Impacts Our Understanding Today

This work did not only concern itself with the cause of bad teeth. Price's unexpected findings were global in their application, and gave insight into the malady of Western society's problems in the early part of the last century. If we follow these studies forward and observe the consequences happening before our very eyes, life-changing conclusions can readily be made. In my own case, as a cancer survivor with months to live, revisiting these truths sitting on my sofa in Del Mar while undergoing chemo in 1986 only confirmed the path I must mimic in order to have clarity, strength, and perhaps even a modicum of health assurance.

Dr. Price is eloquent, succinct and startling:

> While tooth decay has proved to be almost entirely a matter of the nutrition of the individual at the time and prior to the activity of that disease, a group of afflictions have expressed themselves in physical form. These have included facial and dental arch changes, which heretofore, have been accounted for as results of admixtures of different racial stocks. My investigations have revealed that these same divergences from normal are reproduced in all these various racial stocks while the blood is still pure. Indeed, these even develop in those children of the family that are born after the parents adopted the modern nutrition.

> Applying these methods of study to our American families we find readily that a considerable percentage of our families show this same deterioration in the younger members. The percentage of individuals so affected in our American communities in which I have made studies varies through a wide range, usually between 25 percent and 75 percent.

> A certain percentage of this affected group has not only these evidences of physical injury, but also personality disturbances, the most common of which is a lower than normal mental efficiency and acuteness, chiefly observed as so-called mental backwardness, which includes the

group of children in the schools who are unable to keep up with their classmates.

Their IQs are generally lower than normal and they readily develop inferiority complexes growing out of their handicap.

From this group or parallel with it, a certain percentage develops personality disturbances, which have their expression largely in unsocial traits. They include the delinquents who at this time are causing so much trouble and concern. This latter group has been accounted for largely on the basis of some conditioning experiences that developed after the child reached an impressionable age.

My investigations are revealing a physical structural change and therefore, an organic factor, which precedes and underlies these conditioning influences of the environment.

The fact that a government survey has shown that 66 percent of the delinquents who have developed their unsocial or criminal tendencies, strongly emphasizes the urgent necessity that if preventive methods are to be applied these must precede and forestall the primary injury themselves.

While it has been known that certain injuries were directly related to inadequate nutrition of the mother during the formative period of the child, my investigations are revealing evidence that the problem goes back still further to defects in the germ plasms as contributed by the two parents. *(DNA had not been discovered yet – and he still figured this out!)* These injuries therefore are related directly to the physical condition of one or both of these individuals prior to the time that conception took place. *(This validates the theory of "pre-conception nutrition" as a determinant in child development, a concept just acknowl-edged by current science, 70 years later).* A very important phase of my investigations has been the obtaining of information from these various primitive racial groups who were aware that such injuries would occur if the parents were not in excellent physical condition and well nourished. Indeed, in many groups, I found that *the girls were not allowed to be married until after they had had a period of special feeding.* In some tribes a six-month period of special nutrition was required before marriage. An examination of their foods has disclosed special nutritional factors which are utilized for this purpose.

The truth of Weston A. Price's words written in 1938 is haunting. He directly informs us about the future in which we are living. What will the next generations be like? The answers are right here. Price's work shows the genetic variants of the problem, the answers to attention deficit disorder, depression, and aggression seen in our children and us. An alarming number of children are on "behavior" medicines.

Let's extrapolate the information to include society as a whole. Look at the violence depicted in media of all types – the games that children play and the growth of gangs as norms for childhood status and acceptance. Prozac and other mood-elevating types of drugs are prescribed for pre-teens and up to one third of the adult population. IT'S TIME TO WAKE UP AND BE ACCOUNTABLE FOR OUR ACTIONS – This is a bad movie and you're in it!

Correlation to the Chinese Culture

The fact that Price's work is a confirmation of "The Way" would be of no surprise to the Chinese scholar, monk, or family. As an aside, the Chinese took their food with them wherever they were displaced to in the world. I am sure you have tasted Chinese food locally without venturing to China. The same cannot be said for the cuisine of the Outer and Inner Hebrides, Inuit Indians, or Swiss. What we need is a method of physically proving to ourselves where the problem is and then how to set about correcting it. It is for the health and survival of you, your family, and most definitely future generations. This information and method should become commonplace.

Let's look now at some of the cultures that Price studied. Make this your discovery!

The Swiss

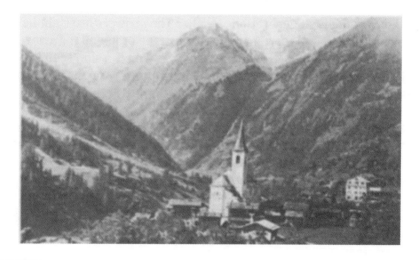

One of Dr. Price's first trips was to an isolated valley system in Switzerland, the Loetschental Valley. Here he found a vibrant people who valued cultural and spiritual values over material artifacts. Due to the steep mountain passes, the only entrance to this area was a small road or path that was buried in snow for many months of the year. At other times, it was treacherous with landslides. The townspeople had no jail, police, physician, or dentist. They did not require them.

Over the centuries, they were occasionally attacked for their prime land and lifestyle, but they easily defeated any attempts to be conquered by use of their terrain, creating landslides to keep out their foe. They were never defeated and for the last 600 years or more, the Swiss in general, marshaled by small stubborn communities like this one, have denied entry to other invading armies.

Hitler himself stated, "The price of entry to Switzerland is too high," meaning the people had superior skill and tenacity in the protection of their cultural and spiritual home. As history tells us, Hitler's armies went around Switzerland. That was a little more than a decade after Price's trip into the area. Eventually, a road was built and in true Swiss fashion, it was a tunnel. Eleven miles of tunnel were needed to liberate or destroy this valley, depending on your view.

Read on to discover the answers to these questions: Are all healthy peoples of the world united by what they eat, how they live, or how diverse and different they are? What is it that they all have in common? (See page 269.) To illustrate these answers, a review of Price's work is foremost. To do this correctly, I will catalogue the food, number of cavities by percentile and special considerations for the group. Then you will see a contrast to the modernized "cousins" and can make a conclusion on your own.

Population Record

Location: Loetschental Valley, Switzerland Year: 1931

Population: approx. 2000 inhabitants

Lifestyle: Farming and dairying; weaving and garment making. No locks on doors. No police, no doctors.

Development of structure: Broad face with wide dental arch, no crowding of teeth seen. Stalwart physical development of men and women.

Quality of teeth: 3 cavities per 100 teeth examined and no toothbrushes used.

Food (Nutrient content): High in vitamins and much higher than commercially available dairy products of Europe or the U.S. at that time.

Special food: Spring butter, stored and used year-round. Used in religious services and used to give homage.

Diet: Slice of whole rye bread with summer-made cheese slice as thick as the bread with fresh raw milk of cow or goat. Meat about once per week.

Contrasting population: Vissoie, about an hour's walk from the isolated village of Ayer. People in Vissoie had consumed modern foods for many years and their teeth proved it: 20.2 cavities per 100 teeth. People in Ayer had a tooth decay incidence of 2.3 cavities per 100 teeth. St. Moritz has a similar physical setting with modern conveniences. Great dental hygiene and education were seen in schools and the tooth decay rate was 29.8 percent. Parents and children who retained their natural diet while living in the town had children who were found to be cavityfree. Vitality was also higher than contemporaries with whom they lived and worked.

Major dietary change: White flour, modern bakery and white flour goods, highly sweetened fruit jams, marmalades, jellies, sugar, and syrups. Traded for cheese and butter products. This resulted in a massive loss of nutrients and increased carbohydrate consumption.

New Understandings from this encounter: Whole heirloom natural grains do not create cavities or create an excessive acidity of the body. Tuberculosis, which was a major epidemic of Europe at this time, was never seen in this population; in fact, there was not one case. When young people went to large cities to work, they lost teeth, and when they returned home to their traditional diet, they had no further cavities or tooth loss.

THE FIRST "SPORTS DRINK" – FRESH CREAM!

Stark observations: Athletes at village competitions were provided with "sports drinks" that were fresh bowls of raw cream!! Where did the idea that saturated fat is bad for one's health come from? These high Swiss mountain villages are where the Swiss Guards of the Vatican are exclusively recruited because they are the strongest men in Europe. This tradition is over 400 years old.

Swiss public health officials considered dental caries and tuberculosis as the #1 health concerns at the beginning of the 1930s. Dr. Rollier of Leysin, Switzerland, was very successful in treating non-pulmonary tuberculosis in his clinic. He had successfully treated over 3500 patients by the time he met Dr. Price. Price ascertained from Rollier that not one person from the high, isolated valleys in Switzerland had ever been to his clinic. Instead, all were from the lower, modernized areas. Clinicians that practised throughout the lower river valleys confirmed this.

Prior to the introduction of modern foods, these areas had supported hearty, vibrant populations, which were then lost over a 50-year period (1880-1930, exactly like the Scottish Highlands).

Dr. Price's conclusions about the Swiss: "The individuals in the modernized districts were found to have widespread tooth decay. Many had facial deformities, dental arch deformities, and skeletal deformities, and were very susceptible to diseases. These conditions were associated with the use of refined cereal flours, a high intake of sweets, canned goods, sweetened fruits, chocolate, and a greatly reduced use of dairy products.

High immunity to dental caries, freedom from dental arch and face deformity, and sturdy physiques with high immunity to disease were all associated with physical isolation and enforced limitation in selection of foods. This resulted in a very liberal use of dairy products and whole-rye bread, in conjunction with plant foods and meat served about once per week." The rye bread was fermented.

Price felt he was onto something akin to the Fountain of Youth, but he also had a feeling that something was not explained fully. In his laboratory, Price found an unidentifiable substance inside the fatty vitamins that was linked to the highest quality dairy products (the Vitamin K family). It seemed to offer some immunity to the ravages of modern society, but what was it? Much like a shadow, he could only see evidence of its real existence. Stalwart with curiosity and purpose, he went in search of another "untouched" population.

Isolated and Modernized Gaelics of the Outer Hebrides

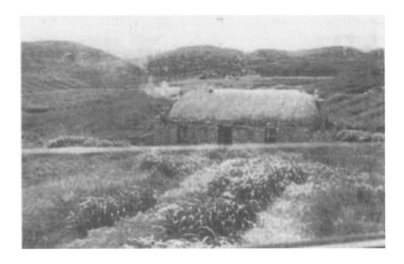

The Hebrides are located off the northwest coast of Scotland. Stories of a superb race of people living in smoke-filled black houses made Dr. Price all the more curious about these hardy folk. When he arrived and surveyed the land, *the contrast to the Swiss could not have been greater.* Gone was the tearful beauty of glacial valleys blessed with the snowline flowers of perennial spring and pristine vistas of contented grazing cows. In fact, the Hebrides were exposed to the full wrath of the North Sea; a more treacherous place on Earth, inhospitable to life, could not be imagined.

The terrain was unthinkable for habitation. Not a tree could be seen except in the innermost regions of the islands. The soil was so poor it would not sustain any roots. Oats could be persuaded to grow. It was the relationship with the thatched roofs that the people had which surprised Price. Peat, containing the rootlets of plant life which grew many centuries before, would grow over most of the isles and in some places, over 20 feet thick. The houses were of earth and had thatched roofs to protect them from the harsh elements.

Dr. Price stated: "Theirs is a land of frequent gales, often sleetridden or enshrouded in penetrating cold fogs. Life is full of meaning for characters that are developed to accept as every day routine, raging seas and piercing blizzards representing the accumulated fury of the treacherous North Atlantic. One marvels at their gentleness, refinement and sweetness of character."

A picture of the life these people lived could not be more different than that of the Swiss, yet these were a very robust and hearty people. The houses were built of stone and earth often five feet thick. Roofs were thatched and heated with the abundant peat. With three rooms and few windows, they often had smoke billowing out of the doors when opened.

This could not be healthy; what was happening here? Price, upon questioning the older inhabitants of the land, was quick to learn that the smoke that impregnated the thatched roofs was indeed integral to the whole process of existence on the isles. Locals knew there was something added to the soil from the recycled thatch, which ensured good growth of the only crop, barley. Every October the roofs were taken down and used as fertilizer on the fields. New roofs were made and the process continued. At this time tuberculosis was also rampant.

Scottish health officials were suspicious of the black houses and made public funds available to "civilize the housing situation." Many times there was a modern house that was situated right next to a traditional house with smoke billow-ing out of doors and windows. No one lived in the older house, but they understood the thatch was part of the cycle and new house or not, there was only one way to get smoke-laden thatch!

Major features of the isles included the scruffy sheep raised for their wool, as it was imperative to have many warm garments in this climate. So tight and fine was the weave that the Isle of Harris became famous for its tweed. Wool and the abundant fish of the North Atlantic were the treasures of this harsh land. The people were a mixture of cottage industrialists or fisher-folk, working either industry dictated by the town they lived in.

The diet was almost devoid of vegetable, dairy products or fruit. It was rich in oats and fish. *A particular breakfast favorite was baked cod's head stuffed with chopped cod liver and oatmeal.* Lobsters, crabs, oysters, and clams were a substantial part of the diet. (A massive Omega 3-rich diet as we will see.)

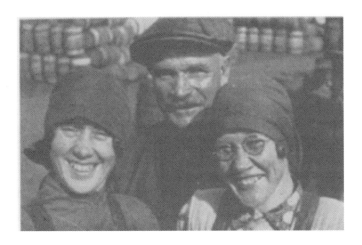

Hearty Islanders with perfect teeth and robust health

The culture of the people was humbling to Price. The fishing village of Stornoway on the Isle of Lewis is the principal port of commerce for the island. On a weekend there might be more than 450 fishing boats in the harbor. As one would expect, Saturday night in a fishing port town would be one of epic debauchery, as the contrast to the harsh environment, it seems would extract an equal pleasure from the soul. Astonished, Price wrote the following about this aspect of Gaelic Life:

> One would expect that in their own seaport town of Stornoway, things would be gay over the weekend, if not boisterous, with between 4000 and 5000 fisher men and seamen on shore-leave from Saturday until midnight Sunday. On Saturday evening, the sidewalks were crowded with happy, carefree people, but no boisterousness and no drinking were to be seen. Sunday, the people went in throngs to their various churches. Before sailors went aboard their crafts on Sunday evenings, they met in bands on the street and on the piers for religious singing and prayers for safety on their next fishing expedition. One could not buy a postage stamp, picture card, or a newspaper, could not hire a taxi, and could not find a place of amusement open on Sunday. Everyone has reverence for the Sabbath day on the Isle of Lewis."

This reverence for a spiritual connection between God, the land, sea, and the people, their humility and gratitude to it, was to be a common trait found in all people Dr. Price met on his expeditions.

Remembering the Gaelic diet had no fruit, vegetables or dairy products, how did the dental health of these people stack up?

Location: On the Isle of Harris in the town of Scalpay.

Population: The remote town of 4,000 inhabitants was on rocky soil and had small patches of soil for pasturage.

Lifestyle: Fishing and cottage crafts associated with weaving.

Development of structure: Excellent physical development of men and women with broad faces and uncrowded teeth. Superb sense of humor and expressive kindness.

Quality of Teeth: 1 cavity per 100 teeth.

Food (Nutrient content): The fish and oats diet was dependent on the consumption of fish heads, livers, scallops, lobster, clam, and cod.

Diet: The people were dependent on oatmeal, porridge, oatcakes and seafood.

Contrasting Populations: Dr. Price traveled to many places in this part of the world looking for isolated pockets of "hearty" people. What he found was sad and confounding. Northern Scotland government officials stated that over the last 50 years (1880-1930), the average height of the Scottish man had decreased four inches and a decrease in immunity to dental caries was observed. A large part of the nutrition was shipped in and included refined flours, canned goods, and sugar.

Back in the Hebrides, Price examined people in their 70s and 80s and found good teeth and few cavities. They told of how the century-old practice of stone-grinding their grains on local mills had been replaced with processed milled flour brought in from afar. On the Isle of Skye where the Dunvegan Clan, a hearty, strong, and proud people built famous castles, the decline was seen in the town of Airth of Sleat. At the school a few years prior to Price's visit, 36 children were examined and not one cavity was found. He went to the town and examined the children and found two distinct groups: one living on modern foods exclusively, and the other primitive foods.

The primitive group had 0.7 cavities per 100 as opposed to the modernized diet of 16.3 per 100, 23 times the amount of the others. A steamboat had recently connected the community on a regular basis with the modern goods, the modern bakery a regular supplier of jams, marmalades, and canned vegetables.

Looking for another "pure" population, Price was disappointed not to find any in the south from Scotland to England. He was alerted to the Island of Bardsey off the northwest coast of Wales where primitive people still might live. When he arrived, he found a people who were the second generation of a repopulation project as the first had been decimated with tuberculosis. Fifty families were relocated to the island to repopulate it. The farmland and sea were fertile, but the land was not being used and the sea was not being fished. The island had a regular supply of sugar, flour, jam, and other processed foods, which displaced their diet. This population was having difficulty with tuberculosis also, and dental caries were at 27.6 percent appearing as early as three years of age.

Conclusions about the Isolated and Modernized Gaelics

Dr. Price concluded that the traditional diet of this area prior to modernized foods built stalwart men and women. Oatmeal porridge with fish products that had some fish organs and eggs were the backbone of the diet and offered immunity to infection, including tuberculosis.

I was beginning to conclude that whatever the traditional diet was, you better not mess with it! *The problem was and is, that we have no tradition!* We are living in an amorphous, cultureless society. We do not eat as our ancestors did, we do not know how to grow our food or prepare our meals. We do not insist on knowing the farmer or cheese maker and the standards of freshness and purity our foods are based on. We eat what is marketed to us as "tasty" and we and our children are addicted.

So we get these results: degenerative diseases including cancer, diabetes, and heart disease taking eight out of ten, with a lifetime of mood and vitality issues along the way. I was beginning to understand just what was necessary to give me a fighting chance to live another six months!

Serious degeneration of the people came from the displacement of the primitive diet with one consisting of white bread, sugar, jams, syrup, chocolate, coffee, some fish without livers, canned vegetables, and eggs. They abandoned the oatcake, oatmeal porridge, and seafood.

From here on, you will find an overview of other populations observed in the 1930s. Price went on to study another 12 populations over the next 12 years. His documentation was eloquent and of the highest scientific standards of the day.

Eskimos

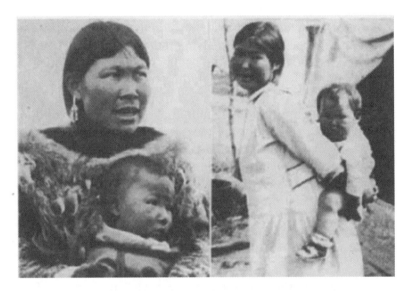

Eskimo women with "2 rows of pearls" for teeth
and children that never cried

The Eskimo was a unique and hearty breed living in winter 10 months per year. Clothed in furs, living off the sea and land there, the Eskimo's diet consisted of seal, whale, salmon, berries, and some grasses. They were very strong and able in the sea with kayaks and spears. The average Eskimo was reported to be able to carry 100 pounds in each hand and 100 pounds with his teeth for a considerable distance!

Price observed Eskimos from Nelson Island on the Bering Sea. This was a group that had almost complete isolation from modern diet. Of 820 teeth examined, he found only one tooth with decay! This is 0.1 percent. On Berthal Island, no cavities were found but two individuals had come from modern diet societies and had 35 percent cavities.

In contrast to Berthal Island, a community of high contact with modern diets was chosen. Holy Cross on the Yukon River lies just above the Arctic Circle. It had regular summer commerce for decades and also had a large Catholic Mission. In the Mission school, Price found one child, who had been raised on a natural diet before coming to the school, that had no cavities. The other children had 18.7 percent tooth decay. Of four individuals who had partial natural diets prior to coming to the school, decay was lower and at 3.5 percent.

The diet of the Eskimo was derived from the sea and land. Seal oil was the mainstay, as they would use it liberally on all foods before drying. Salmon was abundant in the short summer. It was filleted, dunked in seal oil and dried in the sun for use in the winter. Salmon eggs were also prized and dried for use in other times of the year. Berries and certain herbs were collected when available, and the organs and glands of all animals were eaten; these were the superior parts of the animal prized for medicinal properties.

The last thing an Eskimo would want to eat is lean meat. Caribou were always hunted at the time of year when they were the fattest, and a large accumulated fatty strap over the hind of the animal was the best. When they fed the sled dogs lean meat, the type of meat we prize in the modern world, the dogs could not pull the sleds as far and were prone to ill health. In lean times when hunting was poor and the animals themselves were lean, it had ramifications throughout the entire ecosystem and food chain and all suffered. Fat, high in Omega 3 oils not carbohydrates, ruled this environment.

The Eskimo diet is 180 degrees away from modern medical practice of low saturated fat diet with skinless, low-fat meats. When and why did we draw the association between saturated fat and disease? Medically, my research shows that the medical profession didn't endorse a low saturated fat diet. It was popularized by the food industry in the 1950s and 1960s as the modern way to eat.

My observation is that the vegetable oils substituted for saturated fats had a greater effect on poor health than the classic fats eaten by our forefathers. In fact, with the loss of saturated fat, we were becoming malnourished for the first time with losses of Vitamins A, D, and K, three nutrient deficiencies that can have catastrophic effects on preconception, prenatal, and postnatal nutritional development. These fat-soluble vitamins are integral for the absorption of nutrients in the gut itself. So, if you turn down the intake of Vitamins A, D, and K, you down-regulate the absorption of all available nutrients.

Price's observation of crowded teeth with narrow facial bones in the middle and lower third of the skull was universally linked to diet. A diet that was natural had to rely on pure, high-quality foodstuffs. It did not matter if it was with or without vegetables or fruit (carbohydrates). What did matter was that there was a good source of fresh protein, fat, and a fiber source such as a grain.

What is the Diet to Survive?

In a nutshell, in order to survive you have to eat what is locally available. Today it has never been easier or more difficult to eat well. Your wisdom of how to eat comes via marketing and advertising, more than likely? As I said, we have no traditions! When this happens, the link on how to live in accordance to Nature – The Way – is broken. Science and industry can supply ample tonnage to any part of the planet, yet modern society has to utilize the common sense to choose the right foods to consume. As it is human nature to seek comfort and shy away from the pain of exertion, baked codshead and oats easily lost the popularity contest with white bread and sweet jam ending up as the winner. The price: cancer and pain.

It was a double-edged sword, and that sword contained two important facts. Sugars, jams, marmalades, white milled flour, and baked goods were replacing calories of a nutrient-rich primitive diet with foods that were low in nutrients and high in calories. Secondly, without the nutrient-rich diet, a reduction in absorption ability also occurred and compounded the effects of the poor diet. Whether it was the raw summer cheese and spring butter of the Swiss, or the fish eggs and seal oil of the Eskimos, every culture so far had found its own special foods.

In general, Eskimos do not marry those who are not their own race. The Indians of North America were a separate and proud nomadic people also with distinct problems of isolation and invasion from other cultures. With very large geographic and environmental range of living conditions, they adapted – until the White Man arrived.

North American Indians

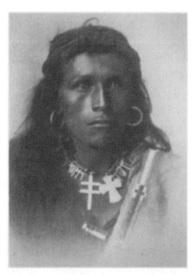

Crossing the Bering Strait over packed ice thousands of years before, the North American Indian had flourished from the jungles of tropical Mexico to the reaches of the Arctic Circle. Perhaps this was the most unique race of people; their ability to successfully adapt to the environment seemed unstoppable. They were strong, proud, and advanced as multiple distinct societies, each which had a unique environment and way of life.

"Primitives" would come to civilization only once or twice per year to trade furs for blankets and ammunition. In the Great Lakes district where the Hudson and James Bay watersheds meet, Price observed Modernized and Primitive Indians. They could not carry back the modern conveniences. Thus, their yearly diets were mainly untouched by the effects of modernization. Modernized Indians were found on reservations that had been set up to provide for the different Indian Tribes: the Mohawks, Onondagas, Cayugas, Senecas, Oneidas, and Delawares that made up the Iroquois Nations.

Another fact of the modernization of diet became apparent in the Indian Tribes of the Canadian Rockies. It was a link between degenerative osteoarthritis and modern foods.

"Investigation of 'natural living' Indians could not document one case of arthritis or physical joint infirmary." Dr. Price said.

However, where the Indian had been in contact with the White Man's diet from birth on, scores of bedridden crippled adults were found. Thus, the development of one of the major diseases of physical degeneration was now firmly linked to diet.

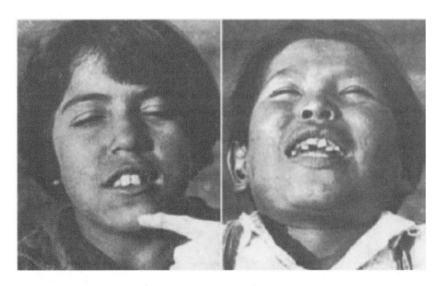

Modernized Mohawk Indians living on White Man's food. Note the crowded teeth, deformities of the sinuses and lower jaw.

For the first time Dr. Price found a group of Modernized Indians that were doing well. These Modernized Indians were a group of Mohawk Indians living in Canada on a reservation. They kept a dairy herd, drank raw milk, had a limited supply of sugar and white flour, and had freshly milled wheat they used for a staple food, bread. People could adapt to their environment!

Price observed and investigated skulls of the ancestors of modern day Swiss, Eskimos, Indians and Peruvians and concluded that structural changes followed when the diet was Westernized, even with as little as one generation.

I can hardly wait for you to see pictures of this. It's true evidence that what Dr. Price discovered and reported was 100 percent true.

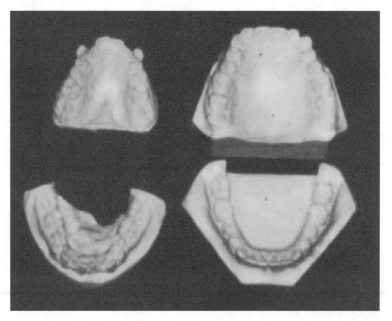

Effects of modern diets (left), on dental bone and tooth formation, compared to primitive diet (right)

ARE THESE YOUR CHILDREN'S TEETH ON THE LEFT?

Structural Changes Seen from Diet Changes

Facial bones

Normal

Wide arch on the upper pallet of the maxilla, all molars uncrowded. Wide lower jaw, resistance to cavities, broad nose and open nasal sinuses.

Abnormal

Crowded teeth, impacted molars, pinched and elongated sinuses, distortion of the sphenoid bone, temporalis, and maxillary muscles. The openings for the cranial nerves exiting the skull were not as round as they had been and showed increased impingement. Ears and the petrous portion of the temporal bone that houses the balance and hearing faculty were underdeveloped leading to increased ear infection in infants and children. Ear grommet operations are the "bread and butter" of pediatric surgical practices in today's society. These changes are due to the parents' pre-conception and pre-natal diets. Lastly, post-natal nutrition that is deficient in healthy fats and proteins reinforces the developmental problems as the child grows.

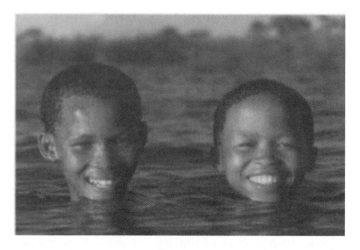

African boys. Note the pinched facial bones (left) and ovoid facial
bones (primitive diet, right).

Pelvic bones

Normal

Oval, wide birth canals appeared to be found with oval
faces. Childbirth was easy and uncomplicated. Women
would deliver their babies unattended and return to villages
to normal activities that same day.

Abnormal

Pinched face with crowded teeth, small jaw and ovoid
appearance seemed to correlate with ovoid pelvic opening and difficult childbirth. (Note: Greater than 30 percent
of children born in the USA need surgical intervention in
delivery.)

Thoracic Cavity

Normal

Wide upper lung regions in the ribcage with shoulders sitting back and good development of chest muscles.

Abnormal

Pinched upper thoracic cavity with smaller air spaces, shoulders rounding forward on smaller frame. Increased tendency towards chest infections and asthma.

Mental Health

Normal

Children in Primitive environments seldom cried, they were strong, very inquisitive, and alert. Adults were happy, peaceful, and had a good sense of humor. Cultures all revered a higher power and lived in harmony with nature and God.

Abnormal

Children were agitated and had uncontrollable outbursts and tantrums. Adults were prone to addictions, poor social skills, and violence. Cultural habits were lost and replaced with modern past times: television, shopping, mood-elevating activities, or escapism drugs like cocaine, meth, and alcohol.

Stark Conclusions

While examining the photos of the boys with the different shaped faces due to different diets, it's an easy way to decipher structural abnormalities in our own population.

The natural diet of the Swiss, Gaelics, Eskimos, and Native American Indians were all high in Vitamins A, D, and the not-yet-discovered Vitamin K1 and K2. The other tribes visited all had similar problems and strengths. The New Zealand Maori were the strongest physical specimens on the planet, pound for pound, yet they could be wiped out by sugar, alcohol, and flour, the same as the Swiss or Mohawk Indians. The balance of fiber, fat, and physical work was also consistent. Elders were robust and vital well into their 80s in these populations.

These societies and the rest of the ones visited by Dr. Price were almost entirely immune to cancer, diabetes, arthritis, heart disease, dementia, depression, and unprovoked violence. All 14 of the primitive groups studied over the 10 years of travel had consistently proved to Dr. Price and the rest of the scientific community – *"modern nutrition causes physical degeneration."*

To Live Now and Die Later, I had to apply what Price was saying to my everyday life, and actually create some time-tested traditions in my own home. Small clues left by Dr. Price's observations of primitive societies were the most substantial proof of modern research yet to be discovered. In the next 75 years, science had found the biochemical explanations for Price's observations. The new Science of Anti-Aging and Lifestyle Medicine had begun to teach them but there was no profit in it, no drugs to sell or procedures to peddle. It has taken us another seven decades to really appreciate the lesson – at the cost of millions of lives lost early to physical degeneration, myself included if I did not change my ways.

The Lifesaving Lifestyle

My health was proof of the serious failure of our system to sustain life. If you have bad health, it's another example of the serious failure of our system to sustain quality of life.

Doctors did not expect me to live past my 34th year. **I learned how to use a "life-saving life-style"** in my personal situation when all seemed lost. Both Dr. Price and his contemporary Professor Gluckman proved that diet before the time of conception is crucial to healthy progeny. The genome has been disassembled right before our eyes and our politicians, businesses, and very fabric of our lives horrifically affected. Once you see the precipitous position we have placed ourselves in as a society and planet, you quickly realize that something has to be done NOW. Just as your ancestors had to fight a beast and win, *you have to survive* fighting *a beast – that of ill health and diet inconveniences – to stay healthy.*

What This Means To You Right Now

Can we as modern people take any useful life-saving information away from this? Yes. Keep your children away from processed foods such as white breads, flours, sugars, jams, spreads, and condiments, and protect their development. Do the same for yourself and protect your immunity. If we use the vision of hindsight and look at our current state of health, we can now see a way out of the morass that will consume our children's children. There is hope, and by living this easily adaptable life with vision and skill, you too can take control of your current health and future health.

CHAPTER ELEVEN
Modern Culture – Exhumed

Digging through the rubble of my life for the last 20 years, the categories of pathology were apparent, and they now had common links to each other. Science was lacing together a universal theory of disease. It put into place a substantial argument for the most common afflictions in society and gave hope for the first time we might have a solution to our suffering. The problem was that the solution was prone to the same resistance encountered by Dr. Price when he published his findings in 1939; it asked people to take responsibility for their actions and to change their lifestyle enough to personally reap the benefit of health!

I am sure that Price was waiting for the profundity of his work to be acknowledged after it was published. He would then work the rest of his life implementing the massive sociological schemes that heralded the lifesaving aspects of his thesis while greatly reducing human suffering. Sadly for all of us, this was not to occur during his lifetime; even with his publication of the most significant scientific work of the century, no one came knocking on his door, excited to rapidly implement his suggestions we now realize in retrospect, there was no money or motive in selling "health"! (Dr. Clarence Cook Little, 1929 Head of Cancer Control Society, 1944 Head of American Cancer Society and 1954 Head of Tobacco Research Council said "it is uneconomic to seek a cure for cancer so we will fund research on the treatment of cancer.") And so it has been ever since!

The Big Conclusion of My Lifetime

My conclusion after 30 years of research, education, and application is that if you want to survive, you must change the culture of how you live, or you will die a slow and painful death. As Yoda prophetically said to young Skywalker, "If you're not frightened now, you will be!"

Today we are well down the pathway of our own demise. Our children are beloved to us and we hope and dream about passing on the mantle of our success to them, but what kind of life will they have when they are sick and deformed? They are unable to reproduce, think clearly, or live without pain in the majority of cases. They are lost on an island of poor health in an ocean of ignorance. By our complacent gullibility, we have ignored Mother Nature and embraced something else – who knows what and in the name of whom?

Perhaps it is in the name of government, commerce, science, and greed. I see not one specific correct answer for everyone. Each person has to be held accountable for his or her own standards. We are responsible for our children and with the completion of the genome mapping project; we are now responsible for our DNA. As difficult as it seems, we must parent ourselves out of the chasm and back into the light of "The Way of Life" that works for each of us. Damming up our molecules with hard-fought science is my only solution to a better future. That's good science, and not the science of food technology.

What We Have Learned from Lifestyle Medicine

Lifestyle Medicine has identified six primary ailments that contribute to the majority of the aging processes. These six conditions affect the lives of eight out of ten of us and will be the cause of early death. They are also mostly diseases created by lifestyle, have common biochemical weaknesses, and are supported by specific traits. We must question our lifestyles and see how we support disease. A close look in the mirror of our own life in full sunlight usually shows a few blemishes rarely seen; it is the most truthful look we can take.

I personally had a germ cell cancer that traveled easily throughout my body. It was taking every bit of available nutrition I had and even cannibalizing my own tissues for energy. My hormonal tests were beginning to show hormones similar to what pregnant women have, because the tumors excreted a hormone called Human Chorionic Gonadotropin (HCG). My body was trying to balance a system gone wild, and the tumors themselves were overcrowding and destroying the very landscape they inhabited.

Cities are crumbling with the cancer of social malice created by generations of malnourishment and worsened by pollution so massive that it's unfathomable. In China air pollution is so bad in some major centers, you cannot see over 200 meters for one third of the year. When compounding the effects of these circumstances on this current generation, we have a horrid look at what we have given our children:

- Rates of obesity approach 60 percent

- Incidences of Attention Deficit Disorder at 30 percent

- Loss of mental acuity proven by declining test scores for the last two decades

- Increases in violence and unconscionable acts

- Increases in substance abuse

- Increases in diabetes up to 3000 percent in some juvenile populations

- Childhood cancer up 35 percent in United Kingdom from 1963-97 and doubling of Leukemia in the last 20 years

From the introduction of processed flour, sugars, jams, marmalades, bakeries, and chemical preservatives, we have created a steady increase in destructive human pathology that is unprecedented in human civilization. From 1347 to 1351, the Black Death, a massive and deadly pandemic swept through Eurasia, killing approximately one third to one half of the population. This incident changed the course of Asian and European history forever. The Black Death was an infectious epidemic that preyed on the weak and malnourished. During that time, most people were weak and malnourished.

Today we have public health methods of control, medications that can cope with the acute phase, and public awareness of illnesses. However, two cases of the Bubonic Plague were reported in the USA in 2006. We are not separate from the past. The exhumed history points its finger at the common plague of the day and finds them to be the diseases of degeneration. Slow, painful death is heaped upon a malnourished population where eight out of ten are now dying from preventable conditions. *You are more than likely one of them. I was.*

Can you imagine your world where food of the highest quality is always available, shelter is no longer an issue, and medical care is attainable but seldom necessary? Chances are you have most of this in place around you without knowing it. Can we stop cancer, diabetes, heart disease, stroke, dementia, and childhood illnesses? I did in myself, and you can within yourself. Can we change our attitude and apply what we know for the benefit of our children? I hope so, as this is the real and "inconvenient truth."

As I look back over a lifetime as a healthcare practitioner, I wonder about the biggest gift ever given to my patients – the ability to think and apply health-promoting, pain-stopping, energy-enhancing tools to daily life. The experience has shown me that it really is difficult to create cancer in a healthy person. To do so, you would have to do many extraordinary things at just the right time. The same is also true for heart disease. If you knew how to create it, would it be easier to defeat?

CHAPTER TWELVE
How Could You Create Disease in Lab Rats?

As you have seen, it is difficult to grow cancer, diabetes, heart disease and autoimmune dysfunction in a primitive and healthy population. In fact, it may be almost impossible.

Modern doctors may argue this fact, saying we did not have the medical knowledge to diagnose the diseases of degeneration back then. Observations of those in the field of forensic pathology put the occurrence of disease at a rate about equal to the rate of tooth decay, which was less than 1 percent. Today we have rates of 37 to 45 percent cancer. How did we do it? If we wanted to create cancer in lab animals, can we support them with the same environment and health-destroying lifestyle, which supports human cancer to equal the same 37 to 45 percent rate of cancer?

What set of circumstances will create the diseases of degeneration almost every time? What are the common traits that seem necessary to carry on good disease development? The British created a 35 percent increase in childhood cancer in just 35 years. Remember, most of our degenerative diseases develop slowly and take a minimum of 5 to 10 years to become clinically noticed. If we had a laboratory, how would we do it? What do we need to know to create disease in our test population of White Man Lab Rats?

The Cancer Challenge: Can We Create It?

To create cancer you need a few consistent things for many months or years prior to getting a body to grow a foreign tissue. In general, 90 percent of cancers are hard tumors with hormone secretion abilities; usually these hormones are estrogens or slightly more advanced glandular tissue. The other types of cancers tend to be proliferative diseases like leukemia and lymphoma. All are deadly and all have a specific formula if they are destined to survive. Here is how to support cancer:

No regular exercise! Cancer is composed of cells with an undying cell line. Cancer is unfortunately immune to a process called apoptosis (the death of a cell). Cancer loves an environment that is anaerobic and low in oxygen. So, if we keep our little white lab rats sedentary without good muscle development or aerobic capacity, that would be a good environment to sustain a cancer cell line. Watching TV or sitting in front of a computer for many hours each day would keep our rats sedentary also.

Tobacco smoke is excellent at reducing antioxidants, reducing cell oxygen levels and stressing out nerve cell communication. It's a proven cancer promoter! As our rats cannot physically smoke we will give them second hand smoke. The great thing about this is that second hand smoke is actually more deadly. The lab will look like a Saturday night blues club.

Reduce sunlight to a minimum and eat a low fat diet. Wear a hoody. We also find increased resistance to cancer when Vitamin D levels are high in the diet, so to support cancer, we need to reduce Vitamin D activation. Nine out of ten of my patients have lower than optimal Vitamin D levels when they start our programs. With less fat in the diet, specifically lard and dairy fat, we can eliminate a good portion of Vitamin D. Next, exposure of the skin to full spectrum sunlight is to be avoided at all costs as it is essential for conversion of the vitamin to the active form. Vitamin D carries calcium to the bone for the building of strong bones and teeth.

Increase insulin levels and free radicals. Take the food supply and refine it, thus removing 90 percent of the free-radical-fighting vitamins, minerals, and antioxidants (SAD, or "Standard American Diet"). Eating 50 to 75 mg per day of fructose, damaging the brain, pancreas and liver as most teenagers do. This will allow a good supply of free radicals. This is essential if we are to maintain pressure on the DNA replication mechanics. A certain degree of statistical failure must be sustained or the system will correct itself. As much as 10 percent of DNA and RNA replication is actually faulty at first pass. The body has a "robot type of corrective system" which tractors up the DNA, pulls it apart, puts in the correct gene and puts the DNA back together. You can call it the DNA police. The DNA police are very good at destroying potential cell-damaging genes, but they have a weak spot we can exploit. The enzyme tractors that move this remarkable system are very fragile and prone to free radical damage.

A synergy of circumstances now works together to increase the odds of developing cancer in our subjects. By lowering the oxygen in the environment, it's more difficult to naturally soak up free radicals. Byreducing the intake of Vitamin D, we have reduced our ability to recyclethose pesky antioxidant vitamins, Vitamins A, E, C and K, which also easily soak up free radicals... Knock one of them out and you'll knock them all out, just like in bowling when you hit the #1 pin!

Create additional free radicals. With the dietary shift to low-fat foods, our little lab rats in our modern day society are eating more pasta, bread, muffins, cookies, and scones. These foods raise the average blood sugar levels, thereby increasing insulin. Insulin is the storage hormone and allows the body to make sugar into fat (usually as a triglyceride).

With an unbalanced amount of starchy sugar in the diet, the pancreas squirts out much more insulin than it normally would. The cells in all tissues become resistant to the effects of constant high insulin, and this begins to create insulin resistance. Measuring our population of rats, we see they are gaining weight. Pushing them into insulin resistance allows a beneficial effect for the cancer cells. With abundant sugar available and high fat stores of low-oxygen-containing sugar, cancer now does very well. Eventually this blood sugar stress creates Type 2 Diabetes in up to 50 percent of our rats by the teenage years. It creates Type 2 Diabetes in almost the entire population that live to about 80 percent of their expected life span. As diabetes is a leading cause of amputations and blindness, we also have up to a 5-fold increase in cancer and heart disease in our diabetic rat. The synergy is fantastic in our quest to develop cancer in our subjects!

Become obese. By sheer random occurrence cancer is the #2 cause of death in modern society at this time, second to heart disease. But these conditions were seldom seen (1 in a 1000) in primitive populations. By maintaining class one or above obesity (BMI >30) the prevalence of cancer is 40 percent greater. If a man's waist measurement is greater than 38 inches or 100 cm, or a woman's waist measurement is 35 inches or 88 cm, the risk of heart attack is doubled. Get out your tape measure. NOW.

Eat a low fiber, low nutrient diet. If we reduce vitamins and minerals from the food supply of our lab rats to trace amounts, this decreases the effectiveness of the immune systems and thereby allows less cancer cells to be detected. Low nutrient, high calorie environments prove to be an effective way of inducing cancer, especially colon cancer; the fourth most common cancer in our lab rats and humans.

Stress emotions often, exhaust adrenal function. One of the most consistent methods to aid the lab rat body's ability to create cancer is to exhaust the adrenal glands. These turbo energy glands are the reasons we can overcome vast amounts of stress and survive. The stress can be emotional and/or physical. The adrenal hormones allow super rat strength when faced with the sink or swim test. One weakness of the adrenal glands is that they are not very good at handling constant low-level stress and will exhaust in just a few weeks. The result is suppression of the immune system and increase in the abnormal sugar metabolism dynamics – a fast track to obesity, insulin resistance, and syndrome X.

We now have a very good method of producing close to 50 percent cancer in our population. Let's recap. We need to control the environment to such an extent we can predict with certainty our lab rats will get cancer.

What Causes Health Problems?

- No regular exercise!
- Smoking cigarettes or smoke passively
- Reduce sunlight, eat a low-fat diet. Wear a hoody.
- Become obese.
- Eat a low fiber, low nutrient diet.
- Stress emotions often and exhaust adrenal function. (Hip-hop music and cool temperatures can do the job as well.)

Results of the Cancer Lifestyle Challenge

We have found some disappointing problems with our system of cancer development. Nine of ten of our test population are unhealthy. Roughly 30 percent of the time, degenerative illnesses develop that do not include cancer. These fall into the following categories:

- Auto-immune diseases, such as lupus, thyroiditis, chronic fatigue, and fibromyalgia

- Degenerative brain diseases like multiple sclerosis (MS), amyotrophic lateral sclerosis (ALS), and Parkinson's Disease

- Coronary artery disease (CAD)

- Diabetes

- Osteoporosis

- Dementia and premature senility and Alzheimer's disease

- ADD and ADHD, anxiety, phobias, and learning difficulties

- Depression

In conclusion, while cancer development is not an exact science, only about 40 percent of our experimental population develops it. The remaining 60 percent will develop heart disease and the other related diseases in descending order. While we are successful most of the time in creating degenerative disease in our test population, we still find resistant individuals about 5 percent of the time. These cell lines can be isolated and moved to the "pro-sports" and rat racing industries.

May it not be a bad side effect to have a population riddled with degenerative diseases? This would serve economic purposes. There's a race going on between cancer and heart disease to see which one wins and takes the most victims. Both diseases and their treatment protocols can be sold to higher institutions. It just may be that it's a lucrative business to develop rats with heart disease. We need to look at how a common and economical system can make both diseases, with elaborate research scams and interventions.

CHAPTER THIRTEEN
How We Create Inflammation, Then Heart Disease

In order to create heart disease, you must understand how it develops. The underlying mechanics of heart disease are straightforward and easy to document. Leading indicators are seen in the doctor's office every day. Yet with our "end point" treatment methods, medicine waits until gross hypertension, diabetes, or obesity sets in to begin a treatment regimen. When pharmacological intervention is used instead of natural methods, it is not long until symptoms prove just how difficult it is to push physiological systems.

For example, as recently as 2006, the American Heart Association had suggested all adults take 81 mg of aspirin per day to reduce the chance of a heart attack. Aspirin is very good at turning off the biochemical pathway of inflammation, which is known to be central in the development of CAD. After a couple of decades of watching this aspirin consumption, we began to notice a high level of pancreatic cancer in those that followed this recommendation. Thus, controlling inflammation medically just became a lot harder. Medicine does not recommend aspirin any more for everyone but it does for those with advanced heart disease. The reason for this is that in those with heart disease that take aspirin, the risk of cancer is outweighed by the risk of death from a heart attack.

Could natural substances do the same thing as aspirin? The Eskimos used fish and seal oil for a thousand years. It became popular as a method of controlling the inflammatory process. In fact, fish oil was more specific than aspirin and had very few side effects other than good skin, clearer thinking, and increased mental agility. If we are to control or promote heart disease, a clear understanding of inflammation is essential.

How Inflammation Happens

To create heart disease, you must have inflammation throughout the entire body. Inflammation pathways in the body are under control of chemicals called prostaglandins. There are three major biochemical pathways in the body where these are produced. These pathways are dependent on a common enzyme pathway called cyclooxygenase (COX) enzymes. There are three basic types of these enzymes: COX 1, COX 2, and COX 3.

The COX 1 and COX 3 enzymes create inflammation and are found abundantly in almost all human tissues. COX 2 compounds, on the other hand, are anti-inflammatory and are attracted to the different tissues in the body via the immune system's chemical and cellular messengers. When necessary, white blood cells called macrophages travel to inflamed tissues, reducing inflammation directly. COX 2 enzymes are called "inducible enzymes" because they become abundant in activated macrophages and other cells at sites of inflammation.

Once the anti-inflammatory response occurs at a tissue, the tissue itself can begin to create its own COX 2 reactions. Every tissue has its own supply of inflammatory agents (COX1 and COX 3) and you need them. For example, if a shark or dog bites you, the tissues affected by the bite have inflammatory cytokines that act immediately to stop the flow of blood and save your life. Next the immune system comes in to stop the inflammation and clean up the site. This is perfect unless your immune system is not doing so well. Heart disease and cancer are products of the body's lack of ability to control inflammation. Lifestyles that are hyper-inflammatory create opportunities for degenerative disease.

It's important to understand how the body does these two most important functions. This is the exact point where diet has a major influence and why heart disease is directly caused by diet in the vast majority of cases. Raising the hands and saying "it's in the family" is only really true in less than 3 percent of cases of heart disease.

Throughout time, man's diet has been variable. The examples Dr. Price, others, and I have used are all drastically different; yet all were balanced with respect to their effects and influence on the prostaglandin system. Did you notice that no matter what the Primitive Diet was, the people were able to maintain balance by having more anti-inflammatory nutrients available than the ones that cause inflammation? These are primarily the omega-3 fats. Specifically, the ratio of omega-6 fats to omega-3 fats was close to a 1:1 ratio.

Our civilized diet has a 5:1 ratio of these fats if we're eating a 'good diet'. Most people though have a ratio of 20:1, or even a 30:1 ratio of these fats and anti-inflammatory nutrients just because they've shifted the quality and types of food. Similarly, the acid/alkaline balance of the diet has shifted to acid and this reduces the ability of COX 2 enzymes to control inflammation.

The unprecedented 20:1 or 30:1 ratio of omega-6 and 9 fats to omega-3 fats yields acid-metabolism that is inflammatory. This ratio is now the norm for modern diets.

These ratios do not allow the white blood cells to mediate the processes of inflammation very well. (down regulation of COX2) As a result, low-level inflammation goes unchecked. We end up with plaque in the arteries; potentiating heart disease, dementia, and stroke.

Today we think about how our food looks and tastes, not what effect it will have on us tomorrow. Ninety percent of food sold in the U.S.

is processed, high in sugar, vegetable fat, and calories, while low in nutrients and fiber. It could be the topic of another book (I suggest - *Fast Food Nation*); suffice it to say, big business and marketing together with farming subsidies of corn and soy products have spawned the industry of cheap foods. (GMO anyone?) We are now playing with genocide of entire generations' future health. The balance of foods, which promote or inhibit inflammation, was close to a 1:1 ratio in "primitive diets."

Small shifts in the diet can be controlled naturally with the immense buffer systems in the human body. But long-term pressure of eating acid-producing foods low in nutrients starts spinning the cycle of vascular decline, which is the hallmark of coronary artery disease (CAD), cerebrovascular disease (CVD), and pulmonary embolism (PE).

How Plaque Forms in the Arteries and Clots Form

With out-of-control inflammatory compounds abundant in our tissues, damage starts to occur, even though it's a low-grade stressor. The artery wall becomes injured from these compounds and cells rush in to repair the irritated area. A fibrous scar forms in the artery wall because the body wants to repair the damage. Small dense LDL molecules and "very low density lipoproteins – VLDL" do this nicely – the type created by the combination of high sugar and vegetable oil diets.

Plaque is also attracted to the site. Plaque is soft and may dislodge and land in another artery or arteriole as a clot. The problem is that the whole inflammatory process is never really halted satisfactorily because our diet is deficient in the nutrients necessary to support our macrophages in their anti-inflammatory response. Once parts of this soft plaque rupture and float into the arteries, they may create a blockage. The body then over-responds to the blockage because it is out of balance. If a clot occurs in one of the coronary arteries, you will have a heart attack. If it happens in the brain, a stroke will result. If it occurs in the leg, (deep vein thrombosis – DVT) the clot may travel to the lung and cause a pulmonary embolism, which can be deadly.

Another alarming point is that in the inflamed arteriole (small arteries) system, this rupture and clotting process is going on most of the time when the person eats a modern diet. Recent research indicates that these microscopic clots travel to the brain where they become lodged. Scarring follows and brain scan shows an appearance of Alzheimer's disease. It is speculated that perhaps half of the suspected Alzheimer's patients are victims of a micro-vascular infarct or "clot." The bottom line is that all are deadly and all are too common.

With rest and periods of better health, the body stabilizes the plaque with fibrin and a hard plaque is created in the vessel wall. This is a much more stable situation and people can live for decades with this. But just because it's stable doesn't mean that negative things aren't happening. Plaque in the vessel walls means a loss of elasticity in those vessels. If the blood vessels do not change shape, they have higher pressure inside them, which places stress on the heart pump. Under stress, the heart enlarges to satisfy peripheral increasing cardiac artery demands, usually increasing blood pressure.

Why People Get Angina

Angina (pain in the heart or chest) occurs when the demands of coronary blood vessels aren't being met. Even simple physical exertion such as walking from one room to another can bring on the pain in the chest, known as angina, when blood cannot carry enough oxygen to the heart muscle. Angina is seen every day in the emergency departments of hospitals around the world and a major side effect of the modern day diet. Usually it's a sign that at least 70 percent of the artery is clogged; only 30 percent of the normal blood flow is left. I think it is remarkable that the body is so clever to not allow us to have any symptoms until we have so little reserve left. Dr. Sinatra, the Cardiologist pointed out to me once that a 10 percent increase in blood vessel diameter increases the flow by 100 percent! Wow!

If severe enough, the low-oxygen environment in the heart tissue can actually cause the tissue to die and no longer beat. Other portions of the heart try to compensate, electrically become confused about the timing of events required for normal cardiac function and the person ends up with flutters, racing heart rates or stoppages (fibrillations, tachycardia, and often sudden death).

Can we predict this in our lab rat population? What can we do to quantify the existence of heart disease? Can we develop any end point control over the process of aggressive, deadly heart disease? Can we predict who and when? These are the big questions to ask.

What Happens When You Take Statins

We are in luck. In just a few short months after starting a balanced diet, high nutrition, and consistent moderate exercise, most of the deadly effects of CAD can be reduced to acceptable levels in the vast majority of cases. When this is not possible and the heart is so overburdened with scarred arteries and lack of oxygen, we can actually sew new arteries into the heart and bypass the old worn-out ones. This is miraculous and many are saved from certain death by this procedure.

We can stabilize the plaque with powerful anti-inflammatory drugs, called statins, which control the levels of fat in the blood necessary to make plaque. This is a last-stage strategy when diet and exercise have proved too little, too late. Just like aspirin though, these statins are not without their side effects. They accelerate the loss of vital nutrients such as Coenzyme Q 10 from heart and muscle tissue throughout the body, shortening people's lifespan by prematurely aging the cells responsible for the spark of life.

The business of heart disease is going well, as these statins are now the number 1 selling medication on the planet (17 billion annual sales 2014). Selling statins is a much better business than the business of chemotherapy. Politicians have actually asked for permission to place these statins in the water supplies of the United States and give them freely to children. It seems that our lab rats need some generational studies to see if this actually will work for healthy hearts. We already know the answer, don't we? Statins are thought to work because of their "anti-inflammatory" effect. Even while limiting the absorption of Vitamins A, D, E, K and others yet unknown. Could this create cancer? Yes, the recent research is questioning the use of statins in all but men who have had one heart attack as being the only risk vs. benefit that is ethical.

Pharmaceutical companies don't emphasize to their customers – the prescribing doctor – the medical fact that half of first-time heart attack victims have normal cholesterol levels. It's these companies that educate frontline doctors who treat these conditions. Fifty percent of the population is prone to heart disease, and yet we have mistakenly linked heart disease to high fat intake and cholesterol levels in the blood. Marketing has created a fear factor to push upon the medical profession and the public the unfounded premise that low-fat diets are the cure to heart health. As a result, in the USA alone, 9 million children under the age of 10 are obese and one quarter of them have signs and symptoms of heart disease, diabetes, or other life-crippling conditions.

While this is alarming and terrifying information to read about, stopping heart disease is as simple as dietary changes and improved awareness. We have demonstrated that to create cancer, you needed a few consistent situations to occur at the same time. All of these were unnatural to the well-fed human.

The Bottom Line on How to Create Heart Disease

The same can be said about creating heart disease. Supply a diet low in saturated fats and the vitamins A, D, E, and K, thereby reducing absorption of the other fat-soluble nutrients. Create a craving for food and satisfy this with high-carbohydrate, high-sugar foods and cheap vegetable oils. Don't forget to add lots of chemically processed salt that bears little resemblance to real salt. What you have here with this type of diet is a marketing miracle, because everyone wants to eat this type of diet. It's a self-perpetuating starvation cycle, satiated by cheap high-profit foods with unlimited shelf life. It will create insulin resistance and leptin resistance; leptin is the mother of all hormones when it comes to turning off the hunger signal. If it's not working you want sugar – now!

What type of success can we expect to have in making CAD, CVD, and PE in our test rats? The good news is that we are even more successful at creating heart disease than cancer; about half of our rats will die from heart disease. Think about it. With almost pinpoint accuracy we can make the coronary arteries clog, clot, and infarct. Many physicians forget that the first myocardial infarct was recorded in the 1930s! By 1960, 500,000 deaths per year were recorded in the USA alone. The lab technicians would be proud of themselves!

To enhance our success in the lab, we need something to weaken our host and make heart disease and cancer more predictable. Bring in diabetes to the rescue! Diabetes alone can create heart disease 500 percent more often than our non-diabetic rats.

What Have We Learned from Our Rats?

The actual death rates from cancer in modern populations are still climbing. The incidence in children is 0.8 percent per year. To the credit of science, remember that these are our best scientists and minds on the planet. We are dying longer. Our "life-span" may be longer in years and months but our "health-span" is not. I believe we need to focus on "Quality of Life"(QOL), as we know not how long any of us have.

Heroic interventions of the medical profession are allowing a longer survival time from diagnosis to death. Many cancers including cancer of the prostate are coined "chronic" cancers, and survival times can go decades – if you can afford the correct care.

Keeping treatment totally devoted to end-stage disease and the treatment of symptoms is ineffective, as the genesis of cancer is predictable 5-10 years in advance if you look to lifestyle, diet, and the acid/alkaline balance of an individual. To date, the recommendations of a diet high in fruits and vegetables, low in vegetable fat, and high in fiber has only received lip service as a cancer prevention method. *We wait far too long to look at our lifestyle and whether it is working for or against us. Your doctor is not trained to ask these questions* about lifestyle and make these speculations as to your ability to create disease until he or she has concrete proof you have objective indicators, i.e., pathology. The International Academy of Prevention Performance and Longevity is now training them to be front line providers of anti-degenerative lifestyle solutions.

Did you know that one of the major benefactors of childhood cancer research and care is a fast food establishment selling high sugar, processed flour, and deep-fried fatty food. **It's insane!** Cancer has reached every strata of the society. I am sure that the Koch family who built the McDonald's Empire has had its fair share of cancer and degenerative disease just like the rest of society. Research has never been funded to look at the missing obvious question Dr. Price or myself have suggested: **People who live in a certain way seem immune to developing cancer. Why?**

Still Looking for One Answer to Cancer?

It is here we depart and return to my personal quest, the same quest as Price and all other serious researchers who value truth in science. The medical model is not working. The war on cancer started in 1971 has been a failure by any measure. We are spending the entire research effort on terminal end point treatment, attempting to reverse the disease without reversing the diseased environment. This is not good medicine and we all deserve better.

Can you see that the culture you live in has many of the factors associated with creating cancer? Is it just possible that by changing the way you eat, your exercise plan, and the thoughts you think could be more powerful and effective in controlling disease than all of medical knowledge combined? Are you aware that forces are at work every day trying to disempower you and abort your attempts at access to high-quality food, vitamins, work environments, or air, keeping you locked in a spiral of accelerated decline?

Silence in Science

The science is clear and understated. The 21st century understanding of degenerative diseases such as cancer, diabetes, heart disease, auto-immune diseases, dementia, arthritis, and osteoporosis now identifies links to diet, at least in part. Because these conditions kill 8 out of 10 people, we now have an understanding of the common elements in all of them. Silent inflammation is silent in presentation. Years, if not decades, go by before the disease is expressed. Silent inflammation works in modern society using the very tools used in our science experiment, where we created cancer and heart disease in our lab rats.

So what's the perfect environment for silent inflammation? Staying out of sunlight, low levels of physical activity, high obesity rates, and low-nutrient foods. Low animal fat consumption, diet high in vegetable fats, high-carbohydrate diets, high refined sugar, and low fiber all conspire together to support cancer and heart disease.

The universal theory of disease has placed the biochemical process of inflammation at the core of both cancer and heart disease.

Heart disease kills one of every two females. Even in first, second and third world countries, heart disease is still the number one killer for the majority of women. With cancer claiming 3-to-4 out of 10 people and heart disease taking 5 of 10, the majority of our effort should be placed on a clear understanding of what these two have in common as predisposing factors and how we can eliminate or reduce these supportive events.

Now that you know your chance of dying of one of these two diseases is eight out of 10 and you know you could beat the odds, what would you be willing to do? *What actions are you willing to take daily, and how much of your resources would you devote to enhancing your quality of life?*

"Take Two Aspirin" Advice is Not Ethical

Information on how to go about reducing inflammation in the body as a central provocative event in the genesis of cancer and heart disease is "the drug" withheld by the medical model. It is withheld because it's not a drug you can buy or they can sell; it involves your choice of non-drug related activities such as food and exercise. The statement or order, "take two aspirin and call me in the morning," is no longer medically ethical in my opinion. Only in circumstances that are the most dire, such as in acute CAD, does aspirin effectively prolong life.

How To Create Diabetes

As a modern society, we are sick, deformed, and dying longer. Chronic disease, managed by powerful medications, yield a low quality of life for many. We have to look at the tremendous resources put in place to combat the effects of physical degeneration.

If we take for granted the basic environmental and lifestyle influences without common sense, we pay the price with the blood of our children. As an example, fluoridation of teeth is a perfect example of "end point" treatment. Dr. Price showed primitive tribes with almost zero cavities, yet cities chlorinate and fluoridate entire populations hoping to keep tooth decay under 30 percent. Antibiotic use has gone rife in the world and now uncontrollable strains of pathogens are immune to drugs. As we have seen, there are populations of people who lived certain ways that did not develop infectious diseases.

In my clinical practice over the last 30 years I have seen a precipitous decline in the health of young people. Problems only seen in the grandparents began showing up in the middle part of life in their children. Today grandchildren show signs of disease similar to parents and grandparents very early in life. There is an overall decline in the vibrancy and collective health of the young people I see – diabetes is a good example of this. As a board certified Chiropractor – those adjustments are not holding like they use to....

Problems Start with Hypoglycemia

When I began practicing in the late 1970s, we were mostly concerned with hypoglycemia, a condition of low blood sugar, leading to tiredness, mood changes, and lack of energy. Side effects of headaches and body pains were additional symptoms related to hypoglycemia. The disorder is very prevalent and anyone who has had a hang over from excess alcohol has experienced low blood sugar.

Hypoglycemia doesn't remain static in the body; it can lead to diabetes. In the 1980s, marked increases in diabetes shocked diabetologists and other health practitioners. It should be stated that hypoglycemia's other medical nickname is "pre-diabetes." In the 1980s, our low blood sugar-challenged population was actually on the rapid pathway to developing diabetes!

The subtle and immediate need to eat cannot be underestimated. Marketers were quick to take advantage of every moment of low willpower. They advertised at traditional "low" times to entice market decisions on sick populations. SNACK FOOD IS NOT A FOOD GROUP! The need to have high carbohydrate snacks in the form of corn, bread, sugary candies, and chocolates, has led to a revolution in eating behavior.

Too Much Sugar in Foods and Beverages

I educate my patients that an average soft drink has about 10 teaspoons of table sugar in it in addition to massive amounts of phosphates, which are acid minerals and affect bone health. The human body has about 2 teaspoons of sugar dissolved into the blood at any one time. Drink the soda pop and you can go into a coma if your pancreas cannot shoot out enough insulin to counteract the intake. It only takes 20 minutes for all of 10 teaspoons to get into the blood. If the pancreas is successful at keeping you alive, it means the insulin has stored the sugar somewhere in the body by converting it to fat while giving you a "buzz" of high blood sugar.

After hearing the 10 teaspoons sugar per soft drink statistics, patients immediately ask, "What about food? Does it do the same thing?" Most highly trained dieticians are told this is true. They create the menus for the poor folks in hospital. Actually I tell my patients that it's not exactly the same. Take an equal amount of sugar from a real food source, say 10 teaspoons of sugar found in two large apples.. Unlike the soda pop, the sugar is not refined, white sterile sugar. Instead, the sugar in apples is bound to fiber, vitamins, and minerals in the apple.

The sugar is incorporated into the apple itself and it must be disassembled from the apple by way of chewing and enzymes in the stomach and small intestine. To release all the energy in the apple, the process takes about two hours. At this rate the slow burn of sugar is handled like a fine scientific instrument – small drops at a time with no immediate danger of coma or overdose on sugar. The apple sugar is burned for energy as the vitamins and minerals necessary to create energy are usually found in perfect amounts in the apple to begin with. The vitamins and minerals needed to metabolize the soda pop usually are robbed from your brain, bone, and liver. This leaves those vital organs depleted and it's a perfect setup for early degeneration.

On Hunger and Cravings

Over a short period of years, the majority of people who eat a processed diet high in carbohydrates and low in fiber and nutrients suffer from the side effects of these choices. Obesity is the outward signal that something is not right, however its much more sinister than that. The fact 50 to 60 percent of the population of America and England are overweight should send a signal of alarm, yet the cravings continue.

When the body wants energy to repair itself, a hunger signal is sent from the brain, creating a feeling in you of hunger. This is fine because you have learned from early years that this signal means find some food. Traditionally over the last 20,000 years, when you ate something it turned off the signal (leptin). Calories in foods had all the necessary nutrients contained in them to "satiate you" and turn off the hunger signal while they nourished you with vitamins and minerals that aided your body in other ways. Of course, there was the odd case of food poisoning that we dealt with. Infectious diseases were not a problem when food was abundant. When life was hard, infectious disease ran rampant.

Lack of Nutrients, "The Addictive Food Cycle"

With our modern diet, calories do not provide enough nutrients to turn off the hunger cycle. In the USA, 90 percent of food sold is processed. Cheap carbohydrates, chemically derived salt, and vegetable fat make up a large portion of the food chain of most modern adults (90% by some USA estimates). Because the carbohydrates in the food do not satiate the body, but only turn on the craving cycle, the individual turns to protein/fat food groups like hamburgers and deep-fried chicken foods that are very cheap to produce further compounding the problem of hydrogenated, free radical-promoting food on top of high starch and sugar intake.

The problem is that eating this food daily changes the metabolism. The serving of crispy chicken just contained an entire day's worth of salt and it was cheaply processed salt at that. Additionally, many of the food additives are addictive which makes us develop cravings for our favorite brand of substandard food units or worse yet, makes us continue eating them and say, "I can't stop eating these."

We think we have weak will power but in reality, it's the sugar and addictive food additives out-competing heroin and cocaine combined for cravings.

Major Nutrients Such as Carbohydrates, Fats, and Proteins are Out of Balance Too

The cycle continues and we rotate to another carbohydrate craving cycle and back to our foods high in fat. At the end of the day we have eaten 20, 30, or even 40 percent more calories than our body needs and received less nutrition than needed to nourish our brains and immune systems. As a result the body becomes agitated, nervous, fatigued, and hyperactive.

Why ADD is Rampant

In children who have over-stimulated nervous systems, we see hyperactivity and attention deficit. This is much the same thing we see in our lab rats when poisoned. The creation of an aberrant energy metabolism from an unending supply of refined carbohydrates and its effects on the brain are now "un-nerving" to the child. Feelings of insecurity, phobias, anxiety, and irrational fears develop. This is the basis for confused violence and aggressive behavior, which is challenging to all who are around it. Teen suicide and juvenile delinquency are rampant in our societies. Dr. Price and I have known for a long time the reasons why. Adult onset diabetes, which is called Type 2 Diabetes, is normally found when people are in their late 40s to early 60s. When I was a medical student, Type 2 Diabetes was called Mature Onset Diabetes and was never reported in anyone under the age of 20. As of this writing, Type 2 Diabetes is one third of the time diagnosed in teenagers and has even been documented as early as 3 years old! Sugar intake is killing the brains of our children! Diabetes has increased some 3,000 percent.

CHAPTER FOURTEEN
Metabolic Syndrome and Why is it Killing Us?

Metabolic Syndrome or Syndrome X is estimated to be in 35 percent of the modern population and another 35 percent are "pre – metabolic syndrome. The body becomes resistant to the energy storage and production demands. Insulin no longer effectively lowers blood sugar and a cluster of clinical symptoms such as hypertension, obesity, high cholesterol, and many other chronic diseases develop. Metabolic Syndrome is a predisposing factor in our big three diseases: diabetes, cancer, and heart disease. With insulin resistance comes inflammation leading to the inability of the body to recover from that inflammation the longer it continues. Asymptomatic pathology is happening: In the arteries, insulin resistance is the basis of arteriosclerosis. In the immune system, insulin resistance can leave the door open for chronic infections to become serious and not heal, irritable bowel syndrome, autoimmune disorders such as lupus, acne rosacea, and lastly, depression. Will the prescription of Prozac actually make any difference at all? Remember Price's observation of happy, cheerful adults who had children that never cried?

We can adapt. We can give our children better chances of health than our parents gave us and hope to return to some assurance of health in our future. This will take much work with constant battling against the market forces of greed and social pressure to conform.

Doesn't Your Child Deserve the Best?

Children in modern society believe they are entitled to a McDonald's Happy Meal from time to time and feel utterly dejected and alienated from "the marketed tribe" if not allowed to share in the kill. Ask any parent of a current day preschooler what type of reception they are met with when trying to persuade the tot to miss a Happy Meal. Tantrums, fits, and utter chaos usually send the parents toward a "feel good alternative" themselves (that glass of wine before dinner, and the ice cream before you get to sleep!) It's the same chemical addiction as heroin – but worse.

We are not that advanced as a society. We are still reliant on centuries of habits, which socially allow us work together. Today, with the modernization and narrow-sightedness of governments and counsels, we build useless, unattractive cities and towns that promise cheap processed foods and activities that require no effort. These "living malls" are the dying zones of our culture. Remember, let's stay out of the sunshine, stay low in vitamin D, and make up for it by eating high vegetable fats. Eat low fiber and high carbohydrates and create the perfect lab rat again. But this time it's not someone else that's affected. This time, it's your children's health and lifestyle. Taking this one step further, can we make a real business of the newly created culture?

Business Model: Mice Or People, You Choose

Our food industry allows us to present our disease-ridden mice (our families) to experimental treatment research facilities (cancer and heart disease drug trials). The researchers believe in a magic bullet, a one-stop "cure" for disease. Governments lobbied by only medical and pharmacy interests insure funding as they try to isolate just one particular factor to inhibit or reverse cancer or heart disease.

Having a genetically weak line of rats, or people, who develop cancer and a system (hospitals screen, classify pathology in the local population, and promote drug trials) that uses "them" for experimentation is a very good business model; sustaining profit for both the supplier of the rats (people) and the researchers that rely on generous grant money to sustain their businesses. It is an industry that feeds itself and sets up ways to justify the supply of laboratory housing, feeding, and screening systems needed for "progress." The "appeal" for charity funding goes on daily. Research may indeed find a magic bullet – but at what cost?

We are reminded just how lucky we are not to be rats! But giving this idea further contemplation we must ask ourselves this: *Are we so sure that we are not the rats?* Scientists can test what gets rid of X or Y cancer for decades. The great understanding scientists provide is the different mechanisms of the cell. Yet with this knowledge, they often create drugs that can halt the cancer lines for only up to five years. Is a five year survival rate really a cure when lifestyle protects 60-80 percent?

Because the cancer-inducing lifestyle for our rats is not changed, the expensive drug uses up its market within a few rounds of chemotherapy. The rats do not tolerate the treatment as they are compromised to begin with, yet we continue in an industry, robust with creativity and grant money. Unfortunately, this is the highest level of technology and sophistication in science that we have achieved in the last half-century. If you're a rat.

When You Change Cancer's Supporting Lifestyle – You Change the Prevalence of Cancer!

I am living proof of the effect of changing the cancer-inducing lifestyle at the same time you treat end-stage cancer. In 1987 when I began chemotherapy, I had but weeks to live. With proper supportive diet, a generous supply of nutraceuticals, and proper rest, my body did what it was designed to do. It healed. **I broke the businesses of cancer therapies by taking responsibility for my environment.** I eliminated processed foods, bad fats, and depression. I made time for exercise, nutrition, and sunlight. I can only compare my experience to leaving the laboratory door open and watching the rats run into the fields for the first time.

Medical research is not to be condemned or abandoned, no matter how harsh my criticism. Our best minds and technologies have created unimaginable advances in humane and well-intended sciences. What I am suggesting is a way to ensure that these great minds and institutions do not fall prey to the very diseases they study. Statistical analysis of research facilities will bear out the fact that they are just as prone to physical degeneration as the average population.

Many of the better educated have chosen to adopt new lifestyles that include more fiber in the diet, some regular exercise, and supplementation with vitamins, minerals, and concentrated plant antioxidants. It's a slow trend back towards Price's fundamentals. This hyper-educated crowd now has created a new demand, counter to the old supply chain and it's called the health food industry. The very name makes a "Stark-comparison" to this other food processing, preserving, packaging industry. But they're all still owned by the same companies. Check out the movie *Fed UP*.

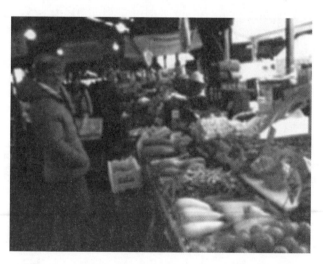

Get up early and start buying local produce – stay away from the Super Markets! Be your own hunter-gatherer.

LIVE NOW – DIE LATER

PART THREE

How to change your health destiny

CHAPTER FIFTEEN

A Stark Reality: How We Die, Heart Disease, Cancer, Diabetes, and Autoimmune Disease.

You are in the midst of a battle. It's a battle that you will die in. At stake is your honor, regarding how you will die. You can die with dignity in your sleep, or be taken down early. As you are now on the field of combat with forces working against you at every moment, it would be wise to understand the enemy's strengths and weaknesses. You do not know if you are face to face with the most highly trained Gladiator on the planet, or a recruit who reluctantly has picked up a sword for the first time. If you know the fighting style, training, and tactics, would you, could you, defend yourself better? Obviously yes, but what action will you make on the battlefield of your life?

Diet, exercise, rest, and stress reduction are potent tools. Combined with accurate and timely medical testing plus nutraceuticals, they make up a hormone-rejuvenating platform that will add life to your years and years to your life! These are your arsenals of self-reliant weapons. Tactics in this fight are the knowledge you have put into action.

What Have You Learned So Far?

You've really learned a lot about health and nutrition, possibly without realizing it. My story is an example of how someone can fight back, find meaning in life, and survive. You learned the history behind why your health was automatically set on the wrong track without your knowledge or your consent. You learned about primitive diets and their benefits and when a diet is considered modern. Lastly, you considered giving yourself a purpose to stay on the planet and work hard on health, knowing that its slow and consistent erosion has challenged everything. Keeping focused on the reasons why you want to stay and fight the fight is the most important medicine you can ever own.

In my own personal investigations, I have found that it does not matter if your doctor told you that you only have three months to live, or that you have diabetes and will go blind or lose a limb. You can simply refuse to lie down and die. Most conditions can be turned around with faith, science, and hard work. Still it's helpful to understand what the challenges will be and how you can overcome them with patience, diligence, and a little self-made luck. You would walk differently in the forest if you knew there were snipers in the trees just waiting to get you in their sights.

CAD: The Most Likely Cause Of Death

It is common knowledge that the number 1 cause of death is Coronary Artery Disease (CAD). There are 60 to 70 million Americans aged 20 to 90 with CAD[1]. Your chance of having a heart attack is linked to diet, lifestyle, and hypovitaminosis (not enough nutrients in your food) but here's the distressing part: Your physician cannot predict, diagnose, or even forecast a heart attack. In an alarming study, Dr. Kuler followed the records of 326 people that died from sudden heart attacks. Of those 326, 86 had been to their doctors (26 percent) within seven days of the terminal event and not one was caught or prevented by the physician.[2]

This might prompt you into taking this seriously enough to act on your own behalf and get on a new heart program NOW. As you learn how to decrease your risk of becoming a statistic, you will gain confidence and functionality in your life, becoming fitter, smarter, and feeling younger. There are many choices to make along the way, and what you think might be your only option, usually is not your only option.

Help or Hype for Managing CAD?

Heroic medicine provides over 170,000 bypass operations per year (at a medical and social cost of close to $100,000 each) in the USA, while Canada and its socialized system opts for exercise, dietary modification, and lifestyle management. If you had a choice between having your chest cracked open like ribs on the Sunday barbecue or changing your lifestyle, the latter is the obvious choice.

Scientific American published a study that showed there was no effect on the second heart attack between the two types of case management.[3] Having the bypass operation did not have any advantage over lifestyle changes when it came to reducing the chance or frequency of a second heart attack. Conservative lifestyle management was just as effective in maintaining the patient until the second heart attack – without the scar.

Technology and Longevity

Facts, concepts, and principles from the fields of Longevity and Vitality Medicine, Anti-Aging Medicine, Age Management Medicine, and Preventative/Rejuvenative Medicine have vastly improved your chances of identifying risk factors years and sometimes decades before you would have an event. Whatever name this new science finally decides on, (Prevention, Performance, and Longevity Medicine is my favorite) it has a real chance of being the most significant improvement in the understanding of how to reduce disease and increase human potential. This leap in understanding comes from the hands of hundreds of years of healers, herbalists, chiropractors, acupuncturists, Vedic doctors, and similar researchers who have looked for the Holy Grail of health.

This is the real deal. In 1986, I bet my life on it!

Now with the new science, a comprehensive review of available research has given real teeth to the tenets of lifestyle preventative medicine.

The hormone theory of aging identifies most of the maladies that have become the hallmarks of modern decay. In less than two decades, we are making improvements in human performance, decreasing and reversing the diseases of aging, and adding to the quality of life with a precision never before available.

Laboratory tests, comprehensive histories, imaging the heart with CT, dietary surveys and genetic testing are all used to protect you from developing heart disease in the first place. Notice we are not talking about a miracle drug that protects you from death. It may be a surprise to learn that James B. Herrick, M.D., reported the first case of CAD in 1912.[4] A contemporary and famous cardiologist of the day, Paul Dudley White, M.D., spent another decade looking for the illusive CAD and as a cardiologist, only discovered three more cases![5]

The Price Was Right!

What Dr. White found actually confirms the suspicions of Dr. Price who was forming his thesis at the same time in history. *"Modern diets are poison to the human being,"*[6] *he said.* Poor teeth are a tell-tale sign of poor nutrition, poor immunity, and lastly a predisposition to heart disease. As we have advanced another 75 years since Price's work, we see the pandemic accelerating across all modernized countries. More people are obese than undernourished on the planet in 2015.

Ron Rothenburg, M.D. and specialist in Emergency and Anti-Aging Medicine states clearly:

> "Traditional Medicine focuses on treating the effects of the aging process while Preventative/Rejuvenate Medicine focuses on treating the causes of aging."[7]

Old Country Habits Die Hard

Those countries that are slow to change from traditional foods are slow to degenerate. We may stereotype the French as being stubborn and spending good money on good food in higher amounts than other "super powers," but look at their results on health. They have the highest standard of medical care in the world and a very high quality of life. Perfect? No. Number 1? Yes.

The USA is trying to break into the top 30! Yet it spends five times as much on health care as any other country. Business is good, unless you want to live well and long. Medical industries such as hospitals, pharmacies, and doctors offices account for 18 percent of the gross domestic product of the USA. England and France, for example, are around 6 percent.

The diet that protects one from heart disease is not so much a combination of special ingredients. Instead the most important part is what foods are not in it. The Stark Diet is a cacophony of great food built around simple rules that promote immunity and do not support heart disease, cancer, and diabetes. Once you understand the rules of diet, you then can adapt the recipes and increase the joy to your palette.

How Male Hormones Relate to Heart Disease

Before you learn what to eat, we need to knock down each of the big risk factors to your personalized heart health and vitality. As a specialist in hormonal health, it was a shock for me to learn that one of the best prognosticators of heart disease for men can be the signs and symptoms of erectile dysfunction (ED). Men who lose the ability to maintain a strong hard erection are also developing heart disease. Think of all the advertisements on television of the slightly graying boomer with the smile on his face when he can now sexually perform for his younger partner, only as a result of his doctor's prescription to increase nitric oxide (NO) uptake and allow for better profusion of blood into the penile artery. Medication does not correct the problem and may make it worse. If corrected in the first year, it can be reversed, via lifestyle alone.

However, if the lack of blood flow continues, permanent damage will occur not only to the penile arteries, but also to the larger coronary arteries. Low testosterone can be a problem, but hardening of the arteries may already be in place. The penile arteries are smaller than the coronary arteries and can lose volume of flow via plaque. It is important to understand blood flow in a woman is similar to men's and lack of arousal, vaginal dryness, and pain during intercourse are the female counterpart to ED. Many times the symptoms of ED have been masked by attempts to control more immediate health problems.

When we think about ED, many people think of the hormone testosterone. Major medications for hypertension, depression, and heart disease affect the brain's ability to produce dopamine and maintain a balance in the hypothalamus. The hypothalamus is the area that stimulates the pituitary to promote gonadotropins. The gonadotropins cause a downstream effect on sexual performance.

Men's sperm counts have declined steadily over the last 50 years, and the nutrients that support male and female hormone production have also declined in the diet to sub-optimal levels.

At my office, I measure your waist and hips, calculate a ratio and tell you about your risk to develop heart disease. As the belly gets bigger, fat around the abdominal organs increases the fastest. It is very poor quality fat, highly oxidized and elevating the bad cholesterol, while at the same time lowering testosterone. Men who have a large belly often have female breasts. We believe they are just overweight; however, their prolactin levels are high along with estrogen levels and thus, this stimulates the growth of male breasts (gynecomastia).

Male athletes with breasts can be seen in the gym when illegal steroids are in use. The hormone prolactin does not break down readily and secondary female characteristics are seen, followed by heart disease and liver disease in this overzealous population. By linking sexual performance to heart disease, we can see the larger picture. The delicate balance of hormones must rely on many factors: diet, an intake of nutrients, and detoxification of by-products, to be successful in this pursuit. This is why lifestyle is the link to unraveling the complexity of health problems.

Both the heart and sex organs have many testosterone receptors. When activated by testosterone, the heart beats more powerfully. Making war or making love both require intensity. (Think about any university football or rugby game you're watching, that's testosterone in action – ggrrrh!) When testosterone is lacking, the players' performance suffers.

One study on boxers showed that the one who lost the match had about half the testosterone level of the winner. Even in close fights, the mental domination had an effect on hormone production and the reaction continued for days after the event. Feel the pump! I wonder what effect attitude had on the great Muhammad Ali's ability. His Parkinson's syndrome was evidence of a complete burnout of serotonin, the other brain hormone that is calming and controlling the motor system. Serotonin is the feel-good hormone, and it must be high and balanced for good testosterone production, otherwise the result is depression and impotence.

Using boxers as an example of primal hormones in action, think about Mike Tyson. He was the one time world heavyweight champion that had quite a sexual history. It was reported he would often have sex three or four times per day during training for a fight.

This is a clear picture of what a healthy heart may be capable of. Sexuality does not have anything to do with mental ability and control however, as Tyson's example sadly points out.

Looking in the Mirror – Marketing to Our Loins

With heart disease taking the lives of 1 in 3 adults and 1 in every 2 women, is it any wonder that Viagra is so popular? Viagra is the mirror image of the problem with our hearts. Marketing to our loins is an emotional G spot, which made pharmaceuticals record profits this last decade and probably in the decade to come.

Women too can have lower testosterone levels. In a woman, the low testosterone levels create loss of libido and vaginal dryness, ending in non-arousal, painful intercourse, and lack of interest in sex. Common medications many times increase prolactin, a hormone released by the pituitary for the production of milk from the female. Men and women on medications that increase prolactin levels do not have interest, sensitivity, or the physical ability to respond to normal stimulation when prolactin levels are high.[8] *This is normal for a breast-feeding mother, not for a businessman on a high blood pressure medication or woman on birth control.*[9] A woman's rate of developing heart disease goes up dramatically after menopause. Estrogen has a protective effect against heart disease. Side effects can have a spiral or cascade of unrelated symptoms and are never addressed by the prescribing physician.

Lactating Men?

So what are we to do? I strongly suggest that you make sure that any medications you are taking have low or no sexual side effects. Do this first because it's not healthy to be chemically neutered! And secondly, it's just not healthy to develop heart disease. There are a few alternatives to the major common drugs. You are responsible for this subtle understanding on how your body is working. If you cannot maintain a strong erection as you once did, look for the cause. If you have vaginal dryness, loss of libido, and are generally moody or depressed, low testosterone and high prolactin may be to blame... not your partner!

Prescription medications are often the first major insult to the hormonal system. With a lifestyle that is suboptimal, heart disease has a great advantage in first world countries where medication rates are high and lifestyles are abnormally stressed. Add to this the fuel of a diet lacking in hormone-stimulating properties and we have an untimely synergy.

Medications account for half of all impotency in men and women.[10] Medication side effects occur via one or all of these mechanisms:

- Direct damage to nerve endings
- Damage to the vascular system
- Damage to the endocrine system

Table 1. Medications that Create Negative Sexual Side Effects

Medications with undesirable sexual side effects on the testosterone production for men and women are included in the table below. These medications hasten or complicate the onset of CAD.

Anti-Hypertensive Contraceptives	Anti-depressants	Tranquilizers	Thyroid Hormone	Steroids	Oral Contra-ceptives
clonidine	clomipramine	chlorpromazine	High T3	testosterones	The pill[11]
reserpine	Fluoxetine	haloperidol	Low T3	Nandrolone decanoate	
methyl-dopa		diazepam		Testosterone	
phenoxybenzamine		chlordiazepoxide		HCG	
propranolol		meprobamate			
hydralazine		Barbiturates (class)			
thiazide					
furosemide					

As you can see, the majority of commonly used drugs in General Practice, Internal Medicine, Cardiology and Urology are on this list. When you need medication, you need it. *The larger question is how did you let yourself get into that situation in the* first *place?*

In my experience, with the exception of infectious diseases, most of these medications are a 10-year precursor of health decline before the physician writes the script. This means symptoms won't show up for at least 10 years. The two exceptions and the most over-prescribed drug of the century are Prozac (Fluoxetine) and lipid-lowering drugs called statins.

Stay Away From Drugs as Much as Possible – Have Regular Sex

There is a link between testosterone and heart disease. With this information, we can also understand that most of the common medications we take for granted will not only decrease sexual performance but are part of the cycle which leads to heart disease. This is your most important lesson, as it has the highest probability to be linked to your cause of death. By being very careful about what medications you use, and limiting them to a medically necessary minimum, you have greatly reduced your chances of creating heart disease. This improves your function on a daily basis and adds to the cycle of life you can enjoy with your family, friends, and business associates.

Having a long and healthy life allows you to support and mentor those around you.

CHAPTER SIXTEEN

Cancer, the Second Reason Why We are Dying

Cancer Trying to Be the Number One Killer

It is a sad comment that cancer rates are increasing. This is not surprising since the US government reports that 90 percent of the modern diet is processed. If we look at cancer with the viewpoint of how to support it, then by mere subtraction of the support system, we can see how to avoid it, or at least reduce the odds of it happening. Building on our discussion on heart disease and testosterone, it should not surprise you to know that breast, prostate, colon, lung, ovarian, and testicular cancer are all symptoms of environmentally induced cancers. Either by diet alone, or by chemical or radiation exposure, we have created a cancer epidemic that targets 1 in 3 people in your life and family. This is not acceptable.

Bowel cancer is the 4th cause of cancer death. This is no surprise as the common highly refined modern diet supports it. It serves as a good example of the relationship between diet and cancer. Science is exactly right when it points to the strong link between diet and bowel cancer and clearly states it is a lifestyle choice to eat right and reduce your risk of bowel cancer.

For the average person, the amount of crude fiber in the diet has been estimated to be as low as 3 grams per day in the diet. Combine this fact with a low nutrient, high saturated fat and hydrogenated fat diet, high in corn and sugar, the obvious outcome is apparent. The minimum amount of fiber you need is 25 to 50 grams a day, but eating sawdust will not help that much, nor will a teaspoon of soluble granules sprinkled over your processed cereal in the morning.

Along with the natural fiber of the two to three kilos (5 to 7 pounds) of fruits and veggies you "should" eat in a normal day, you will get a host of antioxidants rich in constituents that protect the bowel, brain, artery, liver and kidney. A secondary benefit of fiber from natural sources is their ability to decrease bowel transit time. The bowels should move one to three times per day. At this rate the movement of toxins out of the body, bound by the bile salts and other enzymes in a healthy gut, eliminates many potential pathogens. When the bowels slow down, those toxins remain in the body and are stored. Products like Metamucil cannot compete with nature, but the companies that make them argue they are "a convenient alternative in the modern lifestyle."

Chemical exposure is unavoidable and making an effort to maintain a normal bowel transit time helps reduce the risk of all types of cancer by default. Contamination of the human body from prescriptions, food sources such as meat (15 million pounds of antibiotics are put into animals each year in the USA), and estrogen-mimicking compounds (EMCs) such as phytates from plastics, paint fumes, petroleum products, glues, solvents, and auto exhaust, all wildly upset our hormonal system and decrease immunity, leading to an open door for cancer to develop. Most of these chemicals are synthetic in structure and created by companies like Dow Chemical and Monsanto. The human body cannot process them. Synthetic chemicals usually can out-compete natural hormones, nerve receptors, and cell membranes; confusing the signaling and communication between cells. As a result of this, the body tries to adapt.

With phytates, for example, the plastic residue BHP out-competes estrogen receptors. Now this would be acceptable if it just simply moved into place, and then was recycled out of the system, but it does not. Think of a game of rugby or football where a defensive player takes a player on the attacking side out of play. In the real world, he or she gets up, dusts himself off, and gets back in the game. In the world of hormones, it may take a few hours to recycle natural hormones. However, when we play with this new synthetic player (BHP), it blocks the receptors for months to years. It is like the player on the field being taken out for the next five seasons with that position eliminated! Not a fair game, and as you can see by increasing cancer rates, we are losing in every league we join.

It is illogical to think that a human being, exposed to tens of thousands of chemicals on a yearly basis, can have correct hormone communication in the body. In my experience, the body is saying, "My cells are not producing enough hormones because all the receptors are bound. I am not getting any response to the hormones I am making, so I will make more!" After many years of trying to increase hormone production, the glands themselves cannot make more hormones and are exhausted. Nature solves this by allowing or "mutating," extra hormone-producing tissue now called – tumors. Remember, 90 percent of all hard tumors are hormone secreting. (This is the STARK theory of cancer for many.)

Fat Cells Produce Excess Estrogen and Promote Inflammation Everywhere in the Body

Does it start to make sense that obesity is just adding fuel to the fire? With so many chemicals in the modern society you live in, it's easy to pack on the weight to balance a hormonal problem. Clogged receptors from synthetic estrogens in the environment interfere with feedback to glands and organs that produce hormones, thus resulting in massive hormone production. The side effects are hormonal exhaustion, diabetes, insulin resistance, and secondary estrogen dominance, which is created by the fat cells themselves. Is it any wonder that overweight and obese people have a 40-percent higher risk of cancer?

Proper fiber, lower blood sugar, and antioxidant intake may be the only fighting chance we have in binding and eliminating these compounds from the body. These will also help us maintain a proper lean body mass.

With current trends, the following health issues are predicted (see below). Think about your children's world. They will inherit these problems and without the information in this book, have only "average chances to survive" the holocaust created in the 21st century. This is the future:

- Global cancer rates will increase by 50 percent by 2020.[13]

- Men born today will have 3 times the cancer rate of their grandfathers.

- Women with a family history of cancer will have 6 times the incidence of cancer of their grandmothers!

Medicine is the least effective approach to cancer as it waits for cancer to develop before intervention,

- Lifestyle is the most effective defense by my research and experience

- Early detection is second

- Lastly; medical intervention

Is it Alternative or Mandatory?

The Stark Lifestlye and Diet is high in fiber, minerals, and natural antioxidants. These all help to break down and eliminate the barrage of chemical insults we go through each and every day. Revert back to a normal modern diet of 2 to 6 grams of fiber per day as opposed to the 50 - 100 plus grams on my diet and you quickly back up enough toxins to overload the liver. Where do you think the body puts toxic chemicals it cannot remove? Fat! Yep, fat not only looks bad, it's a buffer for your own personal toxic waste dump. Liver first, belly second, hips third. How are you doing?

We have yet to talk about the really bad chemical pollutants like organophosphates and chlorines. DDT, Dioxin, and 2-4 T are just a few you might have heard about. They wreak havoc in your chemistry, as they are synthetic compounds that outstrip your natural electrons, leaving molecules shot up like a cowboy town on a Saturday night! The only chance of quenching these bloodthirsty varmints is having massive amounts of antioxidants available to fight the fight.

It's easy to see how a low fiber, polluted diet can compound any problem we might have. You now see why I have personally taken a handful of antioxidants every day for the last 29 years! We still have to live in a modern world, and I am sure the economy food served on the 13-hour flight from Auckland to Los Angeles is not organic; I want the best possible outcome, so do I starve, or eat the suboptimal nutrition, knowing I have better than average ability to detoxify the nasty bits and still keep my body out of chemical stress? We all have these choices to make and they must be made carefully.

Where The Brown Stuff Hits The Whirly Thing

I personally believe one of the most important vectors of cancer prevention for each individual is bowel transient time. This means your bowels should be moving one to three times per day with good volume, bulk, and color. Yes, they should float also. If you are meeting these requirements, your liver is moving bile and it is purging all the fat-soluble leftovers and sending them out of the body. The other water-soluble by-products such as ammonia go out through the water in the body by urine via the urea cycle. This is how and why we insist on 8 glasses of water per day. (This water can be improved to supercharged ionized alkaline water for added benefits – see Chapter 20)

Dehydration has the following effects:

- Dehydration hampers the liver detoxification pathways.

- Dehydration makes the kidneys filter more toxic material, thus the kidneys are more prone to damage.

- It also makes the blood thicker and more sluggish too, allowing for inflammation and artery diseases to manifest.

- Dehydration reduces lymphatic system volume, thereby making it harder for the immune system to do its job.

Fiber and water have been around as cures for everything from cellulite to depression over the last century. Fiber is part of every cure and part of a preventative and restorative lifestyle. The humorist in the 60s, Shell Silverstein, said quite poetically, "Be on good terms with your arse for it bears you!"

Medical Exams As Prevention Of Cancer

I can argue that the fact-finding examinations done as a routine physical – coronary CT scans or colonoscopies – are too late to be an effective modality. But the sad state of affairs is that you are not going to have a lifestyle consultation with your doctor for another 20 years. This consultation could change your habits to totally sidestep the risks associated with lifestyle. As you are beginning to see some of the most influential things you can do to reduce your cancer risk is to drink good clean water, preferably ionized alkaline water, and eat your fruits, veggies, take your nutraceuticals, exercise, meditate, and use only high-fiber whole non-gluten grains.

If You Miss The Boat, Swim For It!

I can also argue that finding a disease during a medical examination is good practice as the research shows us. The fact that cancer must be present for 5 to 15 years prior to symptoms is alarming, yet if you have not done the basic change in lifestyle work, you will have to go fishing for pathology. If you have a first generation relative that has had cancer, you are at higher risk of getting cancer yourself. In the case of reproductive cancers, and in particular breast cancer, move your medical testing up 5 to 10 years. If your doctor is recommending a mammogram at 45, begin scheduling them at 40. Likewise, consider thermal imaging, an MRI of the breast and or genetic markers to decrease risk and prevent disease from claiming your life.

With symptoms of cancer uncovered by medical testing, the cure rate is only in the low 30th percentile. If I or your doctor performs a "normal physical" and find a bump or a lump and it turns out to be cancer, medically we are in a greatly advantaged situation. My personal reaction is this: "Great, let's get to work!" The early detection of asymptomatic cancer on a routine examination can give us a 50 percent cure rate! Compare the two and you just improved your survival odds by 200 to 400 percent! This is better medicine. In perspective, I still have to say the diet and exercise are still the most influential pieces of the puzzle. But this is a real world scenario, and it happens daily.

Your Colon-Health Connection

The first colon exam is usually done at the age of 50 for men and women. A colonoscopy is not pleasant, however, it too has a great cure rate when asymptomatic disease is uncovered. In the case of bowel cancer, having family members with bowel cancer moves your first test ahead by 5 years. If you have sluggish bowels and a positive history of bowel cancer, move the colonoscopy up another 5 years to 40. Get on the Stark Lifestyle and drink water. You cannot calculate how much you have reduced your chances of cancer when you act proactively.

In the future we will be able to look back and compare those who lived the lifestyle to those who did not, and see the results. *My research at this time is indicating a 60-to-80 percent decrease in cancer for those who are prudent with lifestyle, as we have explained.* This is not radical talk. I think any gastroenterologist would agree with this simple and effective advice. Dr. Price found similar results with dental disease and primitive diets.

Cancer and Hormones

When we relate cancer to hormone levels there is much debate. Looking at testosterone and growth hormone, we find the lowest amounts of cancer when the hormones are highest in the aging population – between 10 and 40 years old. Then when you find a drastic decline in hormones later in life, cancer takes off. Thyroid hormone, testosterone, and growth hormone levels drop, and estrogen levels rise for men and can go up or down for women.

Our premise and that of the American Academy of Anti-Aging Medicine is that the hormone level changes are linked to bad health. In cases where people have tumors that make abnormally high amounts of growth hormone, such as in the case of acromegaly, these people have significantly lower cancer rates than the average population. They do develop other problems, but the main thing to consider is that the cancer-fighting aspect of their immune systems is superior. Keeping your hormones as youthful as possible is smart for reducing your risk of cancer and other age-related declines, too. The combination of increased insulin/blood sugar levels and insulin resistance is now show-ing a predisposition to higher cancer rates. This gives further credence to the points made by many anti-aging physicians, but anyone who has insulin resistance has lost lean muscle mass and gained body fat. Allowing the body to return to normal weight and glucose dynamics (optimal insulin and blood sugar) is paramount to preventing the risk of cancer and heart disease. Pumping iron, doing moderate aerobic work, and cleaning up the cell dynamics give the results of a hugely more productive quality of life.

CANCER HORMONE SET UP

TESTOSTERONE	LOW
GROWTH HORMONE	LOW
THYROID HORMONE	LOW
MALE ESTROGEN	HIGH
FEMALE ESTROGEN	LOW/HIGH*

Cancer And Exercise

One risk factor that does not get the recognition it should with respect to cancer is lack of normal exercise. You would expect that athletes have less cancer, right? Research is starting to show a distinct line in the sand and prove beyond a shadow of a doubt, exercise is pivotal in cancer prevention, and cancer recovery. In Germany, researchers looked at a study of nurses that had under-gone cancer therapy for reproductive system cancers. They asked the nurses questions about their exercise habits. The startling results demonstrated for the first time a significant increase in survival by 40 percent, to the ladies who had moderate exercise for one hour per day during recovery! A 40 percent increase in survival is unheard of!

Improving cancer outcomes was very unexpected; let alone finding a huge shift in survival. This excitement prompted the investigators to look at the incidence of cancer and exercise. Amazingly, they discovered women who exercised one hour per day on average (moderate activity– walking a 3.5 mph or 4 to 5 kph pace) had 40 percent less cancer risk than the average population! As this suggests exercise is one of our best forms of cancer risk reduction. The tipping point being one hour PER DAY, not the 30 minutes recommended.

The theory of how exercise contributes to cancer resistance is pretty straightforward. Exercise reduces insulin levels in the blood. This alone reduces free radical production 50 times lower when ideal levels are obtained. It also burns glucose in the blood, lowering the high levels that can lead to fat production. The lower levels of glucose and insulin contribute to less free radical production, indirectly taking stress off the immune system. Over time, the mechanical movement of exercise, which moves lymphatic flow, and the reduced load of free radicals, raises the overall ability of the body to identify cancer cells and defeat them. Remember the little tractor molecules that go up and down DNA/RNA checking for errors and correcting them every time a cell is replicated and how prone they are to free radical damage? Here is one way of helping this most important function and to do it naturally.

Research suggests that all people harbor cancer cells. Yet not everyone develops cancer. The ability of the immune system to detect and kill unwanted cancer cells relies on a host of interrelated systems. Combine exercise with the Stark Diet, vitamins, antioxidants, minerals, and specific anti-cancer botanicals, and you are now in the right century to reap the benefits of what is possible.

New research has specifically looked into the amount of exercise that has a clinical effect on outcomes of therapy for the most common cancers. As an example, colon cancer, the fourth most common cancer, needs twice the exercise program as breast cancer to markedly alter outcomes. This means that if you want a 40 percent greater chance of survival, you need to be walking or working out well over an hour each and every day. The German study was the first to qualify the relationship with respect to breast cancer and now, recent studies are more specific.

Doctors Katz and Goldman, the founding fathers of anti-aging medicine, suggest this alone *can add 13 to 15 years to your health span*! Dr. Mercola states categorically that the science proves a 14-year increase in health span with just these simple steps. Diet, exercise, supplementation, regular and specific medical testing all become synergistic in reducing risk.

Realistic Approach To Life

The most important thing to know about cancer if you don't have it, is how to avoid ever getting it by a proactive lifestyle. How can regular medical testing ever be successful in finding cancers that have been in situ for 5-15 years when there's been a lifestyle that is pro-cancer, not anti-cancer for decades? Every aspect of the anti-cancer lifestyle must work together, first and foremost mentally handling your stress levels. *What's important is identifying emotional conflict, resolving it, and living with a feeling of hope and optimism,* not fear and helplessness. These emotions have strong effects on your body's ability to produce killer cells that are the scavengers for rogue cancer cells.

Supplying the body with an alkaline tide from a diet high in fruits, vegetables, and antioxidants changes pH from acidic, where cancer cells flourish, to alkaline where cancer cells are generally more susceptible to therapy, and die. Most present-day chemotherapies are very powerful alkaloid compounds.

Exercise (which is alkalizing to the body) is physically necessary to maintain proper body composition, appropriate blood sugar levels, and to physically shake up the lymphatic circulation and keep the bowels moving appropriately. *This ballet dance called "living" is not about getting it right every single day or having to live in fear because you haven't. Instead, it is about being in the "zone" as Dr. Barry Sears would say, letting the body find solutions to internal problems that medicine hasn't even begun to approach.*

I believe that statistically getting it right six days out of seven is enough to maintain appropriate chemistry and physical attributes to protect the majority of people from cancer. This leaves room for the odd night off, birthday, or bar mitzvah along with travel days when you can't exercise. It also allows for the realities of living in a modern world. When you know there is no fear, there is only starting the next morning fresh and brand new. You must remember that your body needs food and water every three hours. The next most important thing would be exercise every other day or every third day but preferably every day.

Exercise is as essential as oxygen. Lastly, because we do not live in a perfect world the use of nutraceuticals is a necessity. To truly be a citizen of the modern world in this new century, you have to be conversant, tackling the issues of cardiovascular disease and cancer. Both of these headless horsemen of death get a 500 percent increase in the presence of diabetes. Thus, diabetes can be a pivotal modifier of risk of developing cancer and CAD. Averting the likelihood of developing diabetes is essential to winning the fight against risk. Therefore, you must be completely up to speed with how to avoid it.

We are all given a brief time to make a difference in this world, and every day is precious. There is no guarantee, just statistical probability; you play your odds. Stark Health Lifestyle protocols may reduce the probability of degenerative illnesses like cancer and heart disease up to 80 percent as we are seeing in our clinical results. Get out and Live Now so you can Die Later with the dignity of a long life lived well!

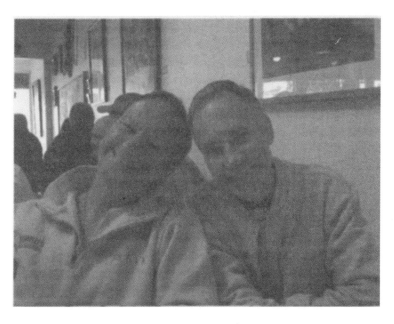

Dr. Davis died in 2009 after a five-year battle with bladder cancer. He was a good friend for 30 years, had a good diet the last 20 years of his life and was a great athlete. Why did he die and not me? The paradox is we do the best we can and do it day to day. Be humble and do it today!

CHAPTER SEVENTEEN
Blood Sugar, Hypoglycemia, & Diabetes

The title of this chapter alone is enough to scare off any self-respecting scientist with the threat of work that will last five full lifetimes! Hypoglycemia and diabetes depend on blood sugar dynamics in the body. Your body constantly interacts with the fuel and food you take in multiple times per day to produce energy. If you get this wrong, your immunity will suffer and silent inflammation will remain undetected, and actively cause harm as quality of life diminishes slowly over decades.

Glucose is Energy

Your body uses the simple sugar glucose for energy. Two hormones control its delivery and storage in the body. The hormone glucagon tells the body to burn glucose. The hormone insulin allows the blood sugar to diffuse into the liver, then the muscles with insulin receptors and store the sugar as glycogen first, and lastly into fat, as a triglyceride which accounts for 60 percent of the energy burned by the heart. Yes, the heart runs on fat! When doctors check your lipid panel, triglyceride is included. Cheating on your diet doesn't make sense because the lab test will tell on you! When triglycerides are elevated, too much sugar and/or alcohol is to blame. Examining blood glucose levels and triglycerides will tell us how much energy is available in your body and what your body is actually doing with it. Simplistically, if you consume more than you need in calories, the excess will float in your blood until it is stored as fat. To high of triglycerides (my ideal is 0.5) and you oxidize the LDL and start heart disease, dementia, and all related chronic diseases, including cancer.

Excess Glucose Is Converted To Fat

Is the problem as simple as moving too little to burn the energy we take in, that energy being cheap carbohydrate? Is this the reason for our epidemic of obesity? This is where the medical fraternities and dietetic sororities differ in their opinions about the quality of those calories recruited from carbohydrates in the diet. High fructose corn syrup, and the liver's inability to handle monumental shifts in our dietary patterns this last century have conspired to make this the pivotal issue in our health care pandemic of obesity and metabolic syndrome.

Secondly, the average American eats about one-half pound (250 grams) of refined sugar every day. If you ask the body to handle this load of (glucose as sucrose and fructose, 55 and 45% respectively) sugar, insulin is called into action to store sugar as fat. But all the fructose can only be handled in the liver. The rate that sterile white refined sugar can get into the body is usually within minutes. Natural food of equal calories can take hours. This sugar dosage places stress on the body's ability to keep a perfectly regulated amount of sugar on hand at all times for your energy needs, and turns the liver to a serious fat globe that will end in "fatty liver" disease or "non-alcoholic fatty degeneration of the liver." Fatigue and exhaustion are classic signs of energy production requirements not being regulated well and tell of a future problem coming.

Consistent overconsumption of sugar/fructose requires the pancreas to produce extra insulin to store that sugar, sometimes four to five times more than normal. With day-in-and-day-out high levels of circulating glucose (sucrose and fructose) and circulating insulin in the blood asking the body to store that sugar, the body begins to ignore or resist the effect of insulin. This is called insulin resistance, metabolic syndrome, or syndrome X, and it shows up as obesity around the middle, high blood pressure, high triglycerides, low HDL, high total cholesterol, and high oxidized LDL-cholesterol.

In particular, LDL-cholesterol conspires to actively promote heart disease and suppress immune system function because it now has small dense LDL particles. This was mentioned before, but sometimes it's good to read it twice to catch the details. Healthy LDL's primary function is to stimulate the immune system via cells called macrophages.

When this process continues over a 5-to-15-year period of time, it sets the body up for diabetes. One by one, the cells of the pancreas are exhausted, never to be replaced. This makes the remaining cells work even harder and the spiral continues to tighten. Diabetics have 5 times the incidence of heart disease as non-diabetics. In diabetics over time, their quality of life decreases. Prior to the onset of changes in our laboratory tests, our physical appearance or actual energy required for day-to-day living comes under threat. Loss of muscle definition, increased body fat around the abdominal organs, and bouts of mental exhaustion as the brain tries to solve the energy problems all come to anti-climax (insulin resistance will drive male hormones down too). Sometimes this is the basis of depression. Other times it sets us up for recurrent infections that wear down our immune systems, leaving us susceptible to cancer, heart disease, autoimmune diseases, and early cognitive decline or senility.

Excess Fat Goes Directly to Fat Storage

We might add that the average overweight American eats about 34 to 37 percent fat in the diet. With sugar in excess and no exercise to turn up the metabolism, almost all fat eaten goes to fat storage and then to sugar if needed for energy. When insulin levels are higher than normal, even protein will go to fat storage. That's why some people will gain weight just by 'looking' at pastries and candies. The Stark Diet asks you to use only the best sources of fat and keep fat down to 20 to 25 percent of your total caloric intake until you body comes back online. If you don't, you'll end up wearing the fat on your fat pads.

It takes a decade or two to get from pre-diabetes or from hypoglycemia, to diabetes and metabolic syndrome. During that time, the immune system is damaged from the free radicals of excess sugar in the blood. The high insulin levels allow higher levels of circulating sugar in the blood to alter red blood cell proteins. These proteins break off raise havoc in all cells. Note, in our historical past as a developing species, this rarely happened. Now these Advanced Glycosylated End Products, aptly named "AGEs," are a great source of free radicals. This leads to immune dysfunction at many levels. In fact, AGEs are some of the worst free radicals the body has to contend with, much worse than normal metabolic toxins (50 times more damaging than other free radicals).

High free-radical levels in the body result from an overload of sugar. The damage is done each time you have high blood sugar levels. The result can eventually be cancer, heart disease, dementia, diabetes complications, and aging. Fat oxidation can also cause a lot of free radicals. Fat oxidation occurs from rancid vegetable oils and hydrogenated fats. This fat oxidation is an insult to the vascular system. Fat oxidation harms the vascular system by turning healthy mast cells into toxic foam cells, which cause hardening of the artery walls.

If we carefully look at our modern-day environment, this is one of the surest pathways to our demise or to our return to health, depending on how you use the information. The Stark Diet gets to the center of this issue; by eating wholesome foods in the right combinations, you end up with simple, clean, slowly released natural sugars from real food. The Stark Diet is rich in fiber, vitamins, minerals, enzymes, phytosterols, antioxidants, esters, tocotrienols, and water.

How the Glycemic Index of Carbohydrates Affects You

The glycemic index of foods gives a quantifiable method of comparison of different carbohydrate foods and how the same amount of a carbohydrate food actually affects blood sugar responses in humans. The types of food eaten and how they release their natural sugars has come under intense investigation these last two decades. Researchers found that the more refined a food is, the higher the glycemic index of that food.

This means that something like jelly beans at a glycemic index of 80 would cause a much higher blood sugar level than a more natural carbohydrate food like lettuce with a Glycemic Index of 15. If the amount of blood sugar released into the blood varies, so does the "storage" hormone insulin and its ability to make food into fat. When you consider good natural foods, they too have individual glycemic indexes and allow one to tailor the "insulin provoking" choices of their diet.

Dates are the sweetest of all at a glycemic index of 103, while cherries come in at a GI of 22. You can see that if you have a very low GI diet naturally, it is impossible for diabetes to take hold; in fact, you can reverse it in many instances with this approach of diet alone in my experience.

The glycemic index does not rate the protein or fat levels of foods; however, some foods that are composed primarily of fat may have carbohydrates in them, such as peanuts. In this case, peanuts will have a glycemic index score closer to zero, provoking little blood sugar response. Researchers also found that the higher the vitamin and mineral content of a food, the slower the rise in blood sugar. Similarly, the lower the vitamin and mineral content of a carbohydrate food, such as in puffed rice products or even popcorn, the higher the food's glycemic index.

The biggest difference between a natural food – one that is unprocessed – and one that is processed is the amount of vitamins, minerals, antioxidants, and medicinal constituents it has in it. Another fact brought to attention by Dr. Royal Lee was this: "Natural foods have a very short window of usability; they rot because of the vitamin and mineral content in them. In order to have a longer shelf life which is desirable if you own a grocery store, you have to make the food less perishable by taking the vitamin-like substances out of the food to make it more stable." (Processing)

Natural foods are loaded with these life-giving substances, and the substances actually aid the body in breaking down and releasing the energy. Processed food requires the same synergistic vitamins, minerals, antioxidants, and other factors to release the energy but it lacks them. Therefore, that processed food must now take these factors out of the body's storage to provide building blocks to sustain the human body. Is it any wonder that processed foods create deficits that can predictably affect our ability to function on a day-to-day basis?

The History of the Glycemic Index

This research on the glycemic index was started in Australia. University students were asked to have fasting blood sugar tested, then given 50 grams of a carbohydrate food, and their blood sugar was measured afterwards. With an average response from a number of volunteers, a glycemic index number was assigned to a food. Not only did this shed light on how we are killing ourselves with high glycemic foods, it demonstrated a way to control our glucose levels with better planning and selection. No longer can we characterize carbohydrates as simple or complex. We have scientific validation that unprocessed foods are superior in protecting the body from diabetes and heart disease. But there are some exceptions when it comes to gluten and whole grains...

Over the last several decades, natural healers and practitioners were giving this dietary advice but very few people were listening. Over the last 30 years, I have seen the health of my patients decline radically in a way never before seen in such a short period of time in recorded history. In my first years of practice, starting in 1980, I saw a lot of hypoglycemia, yet diabetes was rare in my office.

Now, I diagnose one or two new Type 2 Diabetics every month. The acceleration of this is what points to impending doom unless we change our eating habits. Over the last three decades, the Pima Indians have had an increase of childhood diabetes of 3,000 percent! Often it is the indigenous tribe with the least time to properly adapt to new foods that pays the price with their health and dignity.

Knowing the glycemic index of a food is good information and practically a survival skill in today's modern world. But it's not just the glycemic index of a food that must be taken into consideration. *You must also consider the amount of food eaten.* The only missing part of the equation on the Glycemic Index was food density. Some carbohydrate foods were very high in the density of sugars, such as potatoes, while others were not, such as broccoli. Thus, the term, glycemic load, was devised to realistically look at the effects of fiber and actual portions and how energy was being released. The glycemic load finally explains in a scientific quantifiable format why a piece of white bread and a piece of rye bread are different.

With this information we could now single out diets that caused glucose, insulin, and oxidative stress, and those which could reverse, or protect, patients from blood sugar problems. As you might have guessed, the Stark Diet was and still is the most effective blood sugar-controlling diet.

Blood Sugar Disorders are All Too Common

Blood sugar that remains high creates an exponential rise in free radicals "AGEs." These molecular terrorists are the actual mechanism that a diabetic develops damaged kidneys and nerves, cataracts, and infections. As insulin levels rise, free radicals and AGEs make cell membranes incapable of responding to glucose at normal levels and denatures proteins in the body. Once denatured, the proteins cannot function. Thus, a vicious and accelerated cycle of decline can occur to our vision, blood vessels, blood pressure, and immunity. Diabetes is the leading cause of amputations and blindness.

With the availability of *hyper*glycemic foods and a diagnosis of diabetes, pre-diabetes, or active hypoglycemia, the average person's ability to handle the additional stresses in the environment is compromised. Every day another medical report is seen in the popular press claiming that gum disease is linked to heart disease or unresolved infections can lead to cancer; only to confuse and frustrate the average person. But if we look at the mechanism, we can disarm the situation and reclaim an advantage of health and have some clarity, as inflammation is the link that binds all.

Are You Fully Healing?

What happens if you have a severe infection? Of course, you go to your doctor and get a properly prescribed medication to save you from having complications from the infection. Complications can be pretty serious, including anything from scarring of an organ or tissue, to death in the worst-case scenario. It's possible also there could be no long-term damage and complete resolution without medication. We take it for granted that one or two days off work with a handful of antibiotics, steroids, or painkillers will fix the problem. Many people never fully recover from illnesses, becoming chronic.

In my office, I recommend exercise when my patients have energy and feel rested. If they're tired, I recommend rest. If a patient has children suffering from illnesses, I recommend bed-rest for children until they absolutely rebel and must burst out of bed to go play in the sunshine and do what kids do.

The message here is that complete resolution of an illness is necessary, although it is rarely practiced in our hectic society. We send our children back to school not fully recovered so that we may return to work and provide livelihoods for our families. We do the same for ourselves as well; when the major symptoms of our illness have fallen away to an acceptable level, we return to the workplace with a body that is still fighting a lingering illness. Even if your body is only fighting a cold or touch of the flu, it's important to rest, because your body is trying to protect you from pneumonia while at the same time, it must provide energy for the tasks you're asking your body to do.

What is the effect of this cycle of injury and incomplete repair over time? We may feel that we never really catch up, and that there is no hope. Other sinister events, like fatigue, can creep in from vectors we may not expect.

Chronic Fatigue Crept into Doctors' Offices

Thirty years ago, I rarely saw Chronic Fatigue Syndrome. Where did this come from? Why do we suddenly have fatigue as the number 1 reason people go to the doctor? Why are doctors powerless in the allopathic system to do anything but listen and prescribe a mood elevator? In my experience, the downward spiral of health events goes like this: A medication lowers hormone levels as a side effect, the medication then increases the odds of suppressing immunity. Infections now become more frequent. You'll now have symptoms that come and go, ones I call "Rebound Symptoms". This means your body will crave massive amounts of nutrition to correct its imbalances. First you will crave simple energy such as sugar. If you solve this craving incorrectly and eat cheap carbohydrate sources such as refined muffins, jams, jellies, bread, and sweet drinks, you will have immediate energy for an hour or two (Unless you have metabolic syndrome – then you will feel nothing from the food).

Then you will crash, only to awaken or go onto the next round of eating meals with more sustaining food. Your body now craves foods with dense fat that has high nutrients and slow release of energy. Your choices are chocolate, donuts, pastries, French fries, and deep-fried food that is high in salt. Salt helps the adrenals and increases blood pressure.

After a few rounds of this cycle, it becomes a lifestyle!

By continuing to eat foods high in sugar without fiber, you will end up with a 10 to 20 year medical history of one to three new medications per year as your body rebounds in and out of symptoms. This is a true set up for degenerative disease.

The Cascade of Decline

In patient consultations, I find that most have a history of up to a dozen episodes where this has happened in their life. Starting in their twenties, the well-meaning GP is treating symptomatic illnesses. Treating the symptomatic illnesses throughout their thirties; one month it's a respiratory infection, a few months later, it's a urinary tract infection. Next it's constipation and then it's low-grade hypertension as weight gains around the middle.

It's at this point depression is discussed for the first time. That lasts about three months until loss of self-esteem, loss of libido, and time off from work places financial pressures on the family and only compounds "the stress of it all." The well-meaning GP then runs a few tests and says, "All is fine." "You are a little overweight and your blood pressure and blood sugar are well-controlled with medication." "You're just depressed." Now 48, on three medications, you cannot work a full week without staying in bed all weekend, and you do use a little Prozac to cope with it all. You are a victim! Not of your own choosing, but of a system which treats via symptoms, not quality of results. And, if you're female, here comes menopause!

When Do *You* Intervene – Because This is Nuts?

At what point do you take control of your life and act with dignity? Where do you begin with diet, exercise, and mental relaxation as methods to improve and protect yourself? Your doctor is a trained specialist in the identification and treatment of disease. At least six years of study have gone into the expertise necessary to be a good diagnostician of disease. He has taken very few, if any, classes that detail the complexities of prevention, behavior modification, and lifestyle intervention as a method of influencing the development of disease. He has had one class on the pathologic findings of nutritional issues such as anemia, scurvy, and rickets, and that is about it. There are no classes to be taken on the psychological aspect of coaching, motivating, or educating patients effectively to produce positive changes in behavior that advance health.

Allopathic medicine is concerned with the use of medications that have predictable outcomes with acute symptoms. There is no medicine to prescribe when you ask someone to eat, exercise, and rest as a means of disease prevention. Does this make standard medical training obsolete?

Frustrated with his career, the doctor is faced with the dilemma of either doing what doctors are trained to do – writing prescriptions for medications – or teaching his patients. He lacks the acumen to teach his patients effectively about disease prevention as evidenced-based information is withheld from his/her education process.

Your Last Few Years of Lifestyle Choices Determine Your Health Now!

You do not need your doctor's permission to take control of your health! Get naked, look in the mirror, and stand there, taking in the evidence. Do you like what you see? The time you invest in yourself not only shows on the outside, it's happening in every cell in your body.

I once met the famous Olympic running coach Arthur Lydiard, from New Zealand. He told me confidentially, "There are champions everywhere. Become one!"

I believe this is true. That super-fit, tanned, lean, muscular athlete you see every morning on the bike or running down the road as you drive to work is not a god. What he does is normal for him, but not normal for many. Raise the bar on your personal standards. The time, effort, focus, and dedication is what allows your personal form to exist.

Intention + Action = Results!

Many people just let life happen to them. They let their job, relationships, and friends dictate the range of activities they do on a daily basis. They rarely make decisions for their personal greater good and end up as another one of society's normal. They are not only psychologically complacent; they take on all the health risks we have been talking about. Are you like them?

Breaking the disease cycle takes courage, commitment, and personal responsibility. Doctors who look holistically at this problem have to think outside of the norm also. Tests used for the identification of occult pathology must be viewed with sensitivity and as systems or "footprints in the sand," suggestions about a possible trail for an individual to go down *before* pathology takes a foothold.

Three Tests That Predict Diabetes, Cancer, and Heart Disease

The three common tests that predict diabetes, cancer, or heart disease tell a story years in advance. These tests depend on blood sugar metabolism. Doctors who are just looking for signs of pure diabetes as a measure of health do their patients an injustice and do not understand the subtleties of the testing they use. "Normal test results can and do contribute to the development of disease – you need optimal levels and your doctor is unaware of what harm "normal" is doing to the creation of silent illness. Years and decades go by until – OGM I have "......" how did that happen?

Blood sugar is measured immediately when your blood is drawn or when your finger is pricked.

1. **Insulin Levels**

    To test insulin levels, the plasma is used. Insulin must be in the normal range; otherwise, we will die.

2. **Hemoglobin A1c Test (HbA1c)**

    This is the most important test. It actually tells you what your average blood sugar has been during the last three months. In an ideal world, your 3-month blood sugar average should equal your fasting blood sugar levels. The normal range for HbA1c is 4.4 to 6.4 in the USA.

3. **Fasting blood sugar level**

Except the USA, blood sugar is measured on a scale of 3.5 to 6.4. Greater than 6.4 is the diabetic range; blood sugar is measured in mg/DL. Less than 120 mg/DL is non-diabetic, < 4.9 is ideal and US Value is <85 mg/DL..

If your blood sugar level is not ideal, we must look for the cause. Is it the quality of food you're eating? Is it the amount of food you eat? Is it the timing of your meals? All these can shed light on what the future may hold with respect to blood sugar dynamics. You can effectively correct your blood sugar, reduce the level of free radicals, and then the good news happens – you have much less risk of developing diseases associated with low and high blood sugar. Blood sugar dynamics are one of the most important keys to evaluating your health status. Controlling your blood sugar gives you the greatest health advantage and allows you to correct health problems before they develop into full-blown pathology. In this particular sense we contradict ourselves because early testing is truly preventative. We're not just looking for the mere absence of disease we're looking for the subtleties of how your body is working. We compare and contrast your environmental factors of food intake, exercise, genetics and rest. The only "true prevention" then, is the action you take from the information gleaned from this investigation.

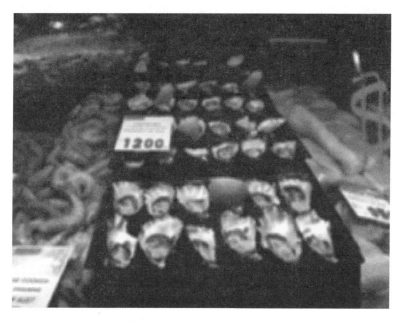

ZERO Glycemic Index, quality protein,
high Omega 3 foods – Yum.
400 gms /1 lb per WEEK is all you need!

CHAPTER EIGHTEEN
Inflammation – The Kingpin When Bowling for Your Life

The Universal Theory of Aging concept coined by Rothenburg tells us that chronic inflammation is the key to most age-related health decline. The chemical effect of inflammation is well documented. Key markers exist which allow us to follow the development of pathology, or the chance of developing pathology. When we look at the effect of lifestyles on them, we begin to see that lifestyle itself is a powerful drug whose effects can be measured in objective laboratory medicine.

NFKB Makes Tumors Grow Wild

Nuclear Factor Kappa Beta, called NFKB, is up-regulated negatively by diet and lifestyle and promotes tumor growth in the body. Simple use of exercise, alkaline dietary foods, and fish oil can greatly inhibit the production of NFKB. Understanding this is vital to the way you live your life. **You can effectively control your daily risk of tumor development by the lifestyle you choose!** Would you agree this is empowering information?

In your environment, you are confronted daily by an inflammatory world. The polluted air, water, and food synergistically work together to set the basis for inflammation in your body. The promotion of NFKB is well documented by these dark, chemical synergists. The better you are at identifying possible sources of inflammation in your food, air, or water, the easier it will be to control the development of chronic disease. We have not even begun to talk about mental influences on the inflammatory process, but we can say that they are substantial. An older, experienced doctor once told me that you have to heal the top two inches first! Good advice; how can anyone heal if their brain is not thinking the right things?

The Sad Story About Osteoporosis

Osteoporosis is an enigma that seems to confuse most clinicians and patients. One in six women who live to the age of 85 will fracture their hip, and one in four of them will die from complications of that fracture within a year. In our society of driving to the mall, parking close to the door so we don't have to exert ourselves, and indulging in all our activities that are convenience-oriented, is it any wonder that our bones are not being preserved? Living longer has some advantages in many ways, but it also causes stress, particularly to the bones and joints. The physiological fact that calcium needs to be brought out of the bone to balance pH seems not to be emphasized – or understood – by current medical practitioners. So you might say, "I have a bone to pick with Osteoporosis."

In the September 2009 issue of New England Journal of Medicine, an interesting article appeared that was called "Increasing Options for the Treatment of Osteoporosis." It was written by Sundeep Khosla, M.D. The article discussed receptor activator NFKB and its role as the molecule that stimulates the resorption of bone by osteoclasts. This was discovered about a decade ago. Again we see a sinister role for NFKB; this time in relation to accelerating bone loss, which is not good.

The article also discussed a new drug in the fight against osteoporosis called Denosumab. This drug can inhibit the NFKB and thereby allows uninhibited bone growth (referred to as an anabolic build-up of bone). What was most interesting was how this therapy compared to the bis-phosphonate protocols that are so popular in the general population. The only anabolic therapy currently in use is a parathormone hormone drug called Teriparatide. But now you can be empowered with this new method to reduce NFKB naturally with a healthy lifestyle!

How You Can Help Your Body Reverse Osteoporosis

Many factors influence the success or failure of the treatment of osteoporosis. Statistics point to the patient being the most unreliable aspect of treatment, with poor compliance. It is my opinion that patients who seek chiropractic care and/or alternative care in general are more highly motivated to achieve a good outcome, and will do well using natural products which induce an anabolic effect.

Products that support hormonal pathways to stimulate bone growth can be used to great effect. One product I use in the clinic is Re-Cal-B manufactured by Nutri-West of Douglas, Wyoming. It contains all the factors necessary for anabolic bone growth stimulation. You will need something like this for yourself to ensure bone health.

What's in Re-Cal-B?

Re-Cal-B is Hydroxyapatite Calcium with Organically Complexed Boron. Each 2 Tablets Supply: Boron (special organic complex) 1 mg, Magnesium (from 400 mg of magnesium chelate) 80 mg, Calcium (from 495 mg calcium chelate/aspartate/gluconate/hydroxy-apatite/ veal bone/citrate) 255.6 mg, Vitamin C 25 mg, Vitamin D-3 50 IU. L-Glutamic Acid HCL 15 mg, Betaine HCL 10 mg, Ammonium Chloride 10 mg, Parathyroid 2 mg, Horse Tail Rush (Shave Grass) (plant,) 25 mg, Calcium Fluoride (Cell Salt), Safflower (flower) Herb 25 mg.) Exercise also inhibits NFKB and has drug-like effects.

Synergistically, using exercise and diet, you have a few powerful tools in your arsenal of health promotion and risk reduction.

Vitamin D is a Calcium Transporter

In calcium metabolism, vitamin D is pivotal in taking calcium from food via the blood and transporting it to the bones. Because we tend to consume a diet that is acidic with processed and refined foods, meat and animal fats, sugar, and vegetable oils that are hydrogenated, we lose the "cofactors" that deposit calcium into bone. Vitamin D is commonly deficient, especially in the aging population, I test almost every patient who comes to my clinic and 90 percent are very low or deficient in vitamin D.

Is Your Salt Naked?

Sodium chloride (NaCl) is the "naked" salt used in most commercial food preparation. Calcium chloride (CaCl) and magnesium chloride (MgCl) accompany sodium chloride in equal amounts in natural sea salt. The undesirable effect of being water-loving makes the calcium and magnesium components yield a lumpy salt. Despite the fact that these are some of the most important nutrients your body needs, they are removed for commercial reasons. In the presence of the factors mentioned above, vitamin B6 and mono-unsaturated fatty acids, such as avocado or olive oil, vitamin D stimulates osteoblasts to produce bone. This can only happen effectively when the pH is correct and all of the metabolically essential cofactor nutrients are available. *Use liberal amounts of natural sea salt every day.*

Cheap Cement?

Pharmaceutical attempts at solving osteoporosis have been to administer highly acidic bis-phosphonates. When these are taken internally, what occurs is the formation of a tight bond of acid and base without any involvement of bone metabolism of new bone. This yields a greater density in the bone matrix, but *this is not a bone-building process* that creates bone with a complex protein/ mineral structure.

Instead, *it is a bone-filling process that can have dire side effects.* In my opinion, it is like filling in live bone with cheap cement. The allopathic doctor argues that this is good enough to affect fracture rates and preserve quality of life. But is it? Spontaneous fracture of the hips and necrosis of the jawbone are two of the more serious side effects of bisphosphonate administration. I believe that the "cheap" bisphosphonate salts are displacing the process of normal osteogenesis by making heavy, dead, brittle bones in our older populations and there are other authors beginning to agree with me.

Good Option for "Good Patients"

When patient compliance is assured, I'm convinced that a natural product, such as "Re-Cal-B" and Vitamin D, will outperform the bisphosphonates.

Those who eat a balanced and varied diet with adequate amounts of vegetables and fruit, in conjunction with regular exercise appropriate for their age, will maintain first and foremost an alkaline pH that allows bone to lay down calcium efficiently.

Second, bone density will be dynamic, not filled with "cheap cement." Instead, the new bone will be provided with all the necessary nutrients for building strong bones. Patients with poor food choices that are deficient in vitamins and minerals and those who have a sedentary lifestyle would not get the same benefit with a nutritional supplement for bone health. If you're a medical professional reading this and you disagree – please enlighten me. I am open to evidence-based science.

Aggressively Conservative

We should take an aggressive stance in the prevention of osteoporosis. A clinician should not wait for statistics from a long-term study. With 1 in 6 females over the age of 75 succumbing to hip fractures and a mortality of 25 percent within the first year, we need immediate decisions and immediate action. Spinal fracture in the geriatric population is also epidemic when compared to third world populations, where a non-refined diet has yielded, by default, greater bone health.

Have confidence that people with a nutrient-dense diet, who exercise often and vigorously, and use optimal supplementation will achieve a desirable outcome time and time again.

Immune System Dysfunction from an Uncommon Source

If we can agree that the average diet is very acidic in the unnatural world we have created, then we can also agree that an abundance of alkaline food is required by the body to physiologically balance itself. Calcium is essential for immune system function; it is literally the most important mineral for the white blood cell. If the white blood cells can't function, neither will your immune system. A body that is acidic strongly supports the creation of inflammation, and this is made possible by the stimulation of NFKB.

Oddly, the majority of estrogen and all cholesterol is anti-inflammatory and helpful to the body. The body knows how to correct inflammation over time, and in the last 20,000 to 30,000 years, the incidence of these two have raised slightly as we age, becoming less efficient. Historically, anyone that lived over the age of 35 was considered aged. This is precisely the age where we see our hormone levels start to rise and fall today, and the cholesterol starts to increase to make more hormones – it's natural.

Say that again!

Cholesterol rises with age as sex hormones that are manufactured from cholesterol compounds begin to fall. Thus, in an attempt to make more testosterone or estrogen, the body asks the liver to produce more base product – cholesterol.

The exception to this natural increase in cholesterol helping out is during the effects of chronic stress when high cortisol levels result in increased blood sugar levels. Long-term adrenal fatigue allows bad LDL-cholesterol to increase and bad estrogen to rise, also. This sets up the basis for heart disease and cancers of the reproductive tract.

You may be wondering how common this is? One person in two will die from heart disease, and about one in seven will die from breast, prostate, and uterine cancers. My colleagues in the anti-aging fraternity are already taking efforts to beat these odds in our patients by testing the specific estrogen ratios and looking at lab tests of total cholesterol fractions, HDL-cholesterol, and LDL-cholesterol.

It is important to understand that osteoporosis begins to really accelerate in women at menopause when 'good' estrogen levels fall. During these menopausal years, doctors prescribe synthetic or horse urine-derived estrogen to women's health programs to allow protection of bone. The risk of developing hormonal cancers is slightly less than the risk of death by fracture, but it is an added risk all the same. Preventing osteoporosis may be just as simple as having the motivation to get enough sunlight and exercise... what do you think?

Paradigm Shift in Medical Studies

New studies that do not rely on prescription medicines are starting to appear in the medical literature. Meanwhile, the debate continues between the pharmaceutical companies that profit from the treatment of osteoporosis and those that advocate common sense approaches that include, sunlight, a good alkaline diet, exercise, and a complete array of vitamins A, D, E, and K, and minerals such as zinc, selenium, boron, magnesium, calcium, and other trace elements. So far, the initial studies are showing superior results without any side effects of cancer, stroke, or gastric upset that are usually associated with the pharmaceutical approaches. As mentioned previously: "Good patients get good results!"

Why Grandma Shrunk as She Got Older

Did you ever wonder why your grandparents shrank in height as they aged? The calcium in their vertebrae was being stripped away and used instead to bolster the immune system and counterbalance the acid-forming diet. Their decreased activity levels further exacerbate the problem. This can be greatly reduced with lifestyle.

One in four women over the age of 75 will have physiological fractures of the spine. This means that they will not have trauma to the spine like jumping off a chair, instead a fracture occurred just from gravity or simple daily activities. Sitting, walking, standing, or lifting a window were enough to crush the vertebrae in their spine. This is not normal aging, it is a pathological problem that can be environmentally controlled via the rudiments of exercise, diet, and spinal health (see a chiropractor, practice yoga).

Yes, the chiropractor can help balance and align the spine of these patients, greatly adding to quality of life. Gentle muscle balancing techniques, low-force manipulation, and rehabilitation all play a role in recovering the quality of life they once had. Medically, a prescription of HRT and Fosamax is the only medical intervention until there is a surgical or life-altering necessity.

In societies such as rural Asia, places where Western medicine is less available, hip fractures and reproductive cancers are uncommon. Women work hard and live long... and they have an alkaline diet. *This is a Stark Fact.*

How to Read Your Bone Density Test Results

The reason osteoporosis is talked about so much is because you can measure bone density very accurately. Radiographic bone density examinations give a clear picture of how you are doing in developing this high-risk condition. Scales are used that compare you to the ideal and to your age group. Comparison to your age group is your "Z" score; comparison to ideal healthy bone is your "T" score. I believe that you should always be measured against the "T" young score; anything else is not normal aging.

Remember that healthy women do not lose bone density! Their bones stay healthy into their older years. Unhealthy populations most certainly do lose bone density. And of course, the unhealthy population is the one we are living in right now. It's the same environment where osteoporosis is now considered a "normal" part of aging.

Digestion plays a major role in the onset of osteoporosis. As we age, our ability to produce enough gastric enzymes decreases, just like the rest of our hormones. Medical textbooks report that the average 50-year-old has 50 percent less stomach acid than a 25-year-old. Yet this 50+ age group is the target market for the antacid pharmaceuticals. Sadly, gastric reflux is almost a given in some cultures. I believe gastric reflux is another indicator of multiple metabolic systems in decline.

The Hidden Truth about Gastric Reflux

I was fortunate to have had a very smart anatomy professor in medical school. He was a Ph.D. in human anatomy, and his thesis was on gastric ulcers and all the associated problems. What he discovered was 180 degrees to what everyone else thought was happening with acid reflux and the ulcerative conditions that followed. Many people, including doctors, still use antacids, proton pump inhibitors, and the like to reduce stomach acid to stop the symptoms of burning and indigestion.

The Helicobacter pylori (H. pylori) bacteria is, in my opinion, not the cause of gastric ulcer but rather a symptom of an opportunistic anaerobic bacteria getting a foothold and not letting go. I advocate taking an antibiotic when indicated, but afterwards it's important to establish a healthy farm of bacteria in the gut with a probiotic for the next six months. I also recommend controlling stomach acid by taking digestive enzymes and eating enzyme-rich foods (live raw foods are such).

As my professor pointed out, what actually happens is that the mucus that protects the gut lining from the ever-present acid, no matter how ineffective it is, is losing the battle. Even low amounts of hydrochloric acid can burn tissue if there is no protection. Research shows a cycle of rebound that occurs when you stop or inhibit acid production. The body senses that the acid levels are falling and pushes hard to make more acid. *Of course, more mucus is produced to protect the gut from the acid.* **This rebound burst of extra mucus, not the inhibition of acid, quells the symptoms of reflux.**

Over time, this whipping of the gastric lining exhausts the mucus-forming cells and then causes erosion and ulcers. Oddly, when I was a boy and gastric ulcer was common in alcoholics, drinking a milk diet was the cure of the day... Mucus anyone?

The next physiological fact that occurs is with the lower amounts of stomach acid: protein is not broken down quickly enough. If you put white flour, sugar, and yeast together you get bubbles. The best place to put the bowl is on top the refrigerator which is about the same temperature as your stomach... but no hotter. At the temperature of 36 to 37 degrees C (98.6F), fermentation of simple sugars occurs in minutes in the stomach because the stomach slows its transit time (emptying time) to deal with inefficient digestion, therefore gas and bloating occur, pushing on the gastric contents and organs.

You have a tissue at the bottom of the esophagus strategically located at a spot where mucus cannot protect it from the stomach acid. A gas bubble stretching and dilating the opening can be very painful. The stomach only has a single type of nerve fiber to record pain, one called stretch fibers.

When gastric muscle fibers balloon out with gas distention, the nerve fibers inside the muscle send a message of pain that can send a person to the emergency room with heart attack-like symptoms. Several of my patients have told me their story about how they were almost scheduled for a life-saving bypass surgery when the Gaviscon or Losec medications prescribed for their gastric upset were finally detected as the problem!

When the protein you eat is not broken down efficiently, you start to lose the ability to absorb not only the amino acids, but also the vitamins, enzymes, and antioxidants from food. Many people start to shy away from heavier protein foods as they associate them with creating gut pain. By reducing protein and increasing carbohydrates, we now have the enigma of geriatric hypo-nutrition, and it's stressing the blood sugar, accelerating the aging process.

How Your Stomach Works

The digestive tract has three basic parts: the stomach, the small intestine, and the large intestine. If the digestion in the stomach is off, then the pH and synergy of contents from the upper gastric area do not help the lower one. It actually makes the process of digestion more difficult in the parts lower on down the tract. With increases in gas and bloating and generally poor digestion, friendly bacteria in the wrong environment can mutate into unhealthy bacteria and cause illness. These strains can be gas-forming and toxic to the digestive tissues and nerves anywhere in the body.

On a modern 90 percent-processed food diet, fuel is abundant in the form of cheap carbohydrates and poorly digested protein for the formation of some very nasty gut problems. Remember that bowel cancer is the fourth leading cause of cancer death; now you know why. There is still more to the story and it will not only relate to osteoporosis but to a host of other modern diseases.

After digestive power is lost and protective stomach mucus is reduced by stress and poor food choices, there's a downward spiral of events that lead to the devitalized existence common in so many people. I teach doctors to treat digestion first by correcting pH, which stops the complex cycle of digestive degeneration. Once digestion is off, our ability to build bone or support any other function is greatly compromised. It can take decades to show as pathology.

How the Immune System Interacts with Your Digestive System

Our immune system surrounds the gut. The gut can actually use 70 percent of the immune system's resources to protect and deal with the toxic, sore, and unstable digestion, leaving other areas in the body to go into faster decline or accelerated aging. Imagine what happens when you have a sore throat with swollen tonsils and adenoids creating a very difficult time swallowing. Now, imagine that you have at least 27 feet of small intestine with that going on! Many patients, when this is explained to them, reply that yes, that is what it feels like.

The next issue is about the junctions between the cells that join together; holding hands so to speak, to form this 10-meter tube that keeps the outside world outside until it's broken down. Those cells are bound together with a very unique and especially tough material to make what are called "tight junctions" between the cells. These are almost impossible to break apart. And that is a good thing, because the blood supply is just on the other side of the fence!

There are only three things that can break the "tight junctions" and as you would expect the body has a violent reaction to "leaks" in its wall. It will have a massive inflammatory response, followed by a proper flush of the area will all the water it can manage. In other words, you get explosive diarrhea and blood loss. And what are these offending agents?

Cholera, Diptheria, and the gluten proteins, glutenin and glieden. The first two are not-so-common fecal contamination-borne infectious diseases – but the third is in two thirds of the food you eat on a daily basis. The most severe form is called celiac disease and effects about 2 percent of the population. The second variation of glutinen and glieden sensitivity affects everyone else. Recent research has shown seven distinct sub-proteins of glieden that can break tight junctions. Only 50 percent of those people have digestive problems. The rest can cause anything from epileptic fits and dementia, to autoimmune disorders such as multiple sclerosis, Parkinson's disease, and thyroiditis to name just a few. It is a pandemic of global proportions. Now undigested food and other materials can get through into the blood where the show really begins.

The immune system has an absolute fit over undigested protein. Undigested proteins clearly resemble something unknown to the body that may threaten the survival of the host – you! Knowing that about 70 percent of your immune system's activities are devoted to assist your digestive system, what do you do when under stress? With weeks, months, and even years of poor digestion and the average selection of modern food that goes along with that, you have an immune system under siege!

What Happens When There's Undigested Food in the Gut?

The body will build defenses to invading proteins, not only the gluten, but other things that just happen to be in the meal, like undigested eggs, milk, soy and corn, just like it does to harmful bacteria. Normally, in a healthy individual the battle will last a few days to a couple of weeks at most. Then digestive power returns and brings energy along with it. Lastly, stamina returns.

But we keep eating gluten products and instigating the inflammation. Our modern-day habit is to grab a quick bite, gulp down a cornor soy-based sugary drink, and take the well-advertised indigestion/cold/flu/cough medicine to suppress your body's healing symptoms, and you now have the basis for allergies that start in the digestive tract and move right through the body to produce lowered immunity and increased inflammation, which is the perfect set-up for cancer, diabetes, heart disease, autoimmune disorders, dementia, and now osteoporosis.

Digesting what's been said: Eat slowly, use enzymes, take supplements, never eat when feeling upset, drink 8 to 10 glasses of water a day, and by all means drop all gluten products from your diet – forever!

In review of how digestion can start the cycle of degenerative disease: Low stomach acid caused by chronic poor eating, emotional stress, or all three, allow gut pH to decrease the ability to digest your foods. This will hasten "leaky gut syndrome" also. Maintaining proper bacterial flora is very difficult in a low fiber, high carbohydrate, and poorly digested protein environment. Friendly bacteria make vitamins but now, with poorly digested protein and an improper pH environment in the stomach, small intestine, and colon, their levels decrease. This, in turn, now affects your ability to absorb and bind calcium and other essential minerals, including the fat-soluble vitamins.

Natural killer cells now shift to fighting foreign proteins getting into the blood via broken tight junctions (leaky gut). Seventy percent of the body's immune system is devoted to activities in the digestive tract trying to fight a battle against your diet and sometimes your own damaged cell fragments (the beginning of autoimmune disorders). This is instead of aiding your immune-surveillance system by picking up the odd rogue cancer cell or abnormal bug that gets past the post. How do we stop this rampant decay of vitality and spirit brought about by cheap food, high sugar, and wheat? We need to look for examples where it does not occur in our modern world.

Why French People Stay Healthy Longer – Most of the Time

The French Paradox makes more sense when you consider how taking twice as long to eat can dramatically improve your chances that you don't develop heart disease, cancer, and osteoporosis. Research in the 1970s uncovered the fact that the French have less heart disease than all of their European cousins even when their total cholesterol levels said they should have the same amount. Many theories were put forward as to why this was true – maybe it was food quality, wine, or attitude, but all these were debunked until a few years ago. For example, when Norwegians were given the French diet, they did a little better on heart attack rates, but still didn't come anywhere close to the statistics of the French. So, it was not the food specifically.

Eat Slow in Good Company

Looking at the social network involved with eating, it became obvious that the French took exactly twice as long to eat as the rest of Europe! The French sat at the table for 40 minutes, while the rest of us cleaned the table 20 minutes later. My digestive theory was proven right. By slower eating, you had mechanically more time to chemically break down food in the mouth. Eating slower also meant you might actually enjoy the people around the table; it might actually mean there was a table!

With better nutrient absorption, you have better immunity and less inflammation, and so lower rates of degenerative disease including heart disease and cancer. Doubling your eating time may actually give better results than those offered from statin and antacid drugs combined! No side effects either, except in your productivity and longevity.

What the Farmers can teach us:

Remember the farmers who could not keep as high stock units on the farm when they dropped the use of chemicals and went organic? It took as little as one year to see results of increased fertility and decreased disease. David Crutchley, a Central Otago sheep farmer in New Zealand, used bio-intensive methods on his paddocks for and went from 1.3 lambs per ewe to 2.0 in just three years! He also tripled his profits, had less disease, and fourteen percent more meat on the bone. What was most amazing though was the Omega 3 to Omega 6 ratio in the meat. It was now 1:1. This meant you could have more anti-inflammatory Omega 3 from a piece of David's lamb than you could from a farm raised salmon! U.S . feedlot beef will have ratios of 25:1 or more. This is the equivalent of eating a pro-inflammatory, acid gut bomb! Sore joints anyone?

Bowel and reproductive system cancers are less frequent in France than other European countries and the USA. You cannot just take calcium to correct osteoporosis. You need sunlight for vitamin D to aid the bacteria in the gut to produce and help absorb vitamins K and K2. You must greatly increase absorption of vitamin E and vitamin A, two nutrients essential to hormone production and immune function. Without this kick-start, there is little hope of halting osteoporosis medically without creating other problems. We now see why French people who eat a high fat, high cholesterol diet have the lowest heart disease rate in Europe: high quality food and quality time taken to eat it.

The Best Osteoporosis Prevention Strategy

The first drug of choice that doctor SHOULD give patients with suspected or occult osteoporosis is hydrochloric acid. The good doctors should then throw in a prescription for a good dose of sunshine. Symptomatically, this is much more effective than antacids, and in the long term it corrects the problem by taking stress off the digestive pH. This strategy allows mucus to accumulate, better protecting the gut wall. This in turn leads to more beneficial bacterial colonies at the right pH that aid in the absorption of minerals, especially calcium. This "top down approach" of getting digestive pH right and asking for a little help from the patient in terms of lifestyle management is a very prudent approach to the prevention of osteoporosis, with multiple vectors of benefit.

Dementia and autoimmune-related diseases are linked to wheat, gut pH, and the body's inability to cope with a low-fat high-carb diet. Mild cognitive impairment, pre-senile dementia, dementia and Alzheimer's disease are all on the rise. Mild cognitive impairment starts to become apparent in the late 50s and early 60s. Usually, it is a symptom of arteriosclerosis and reduced blood supply to the higher centers of the brain.

Brain Pathologies Start from the Same Process as Heart Disease

Our short-term memory center, the amygdala, is one of the most active areas in the brain. Short-term memory function is essential to our survival and our observation of the environment. Therefore, it can quickly become problematic and its results are easy to recognize by family and friends. The chemical pathology of amyloidosis as seen in Alzheimer's disease, multiple sclerosis, Parkinson's disease, and dementia is, in my opinion, a reflection of an ineffective immune system response stemming from the lifestyle. It's similar to the scar tissue found in the arterial walls with narrowed diameter and reduced blood flow. The scar tissue created in the central nervous system (CNS) is a byproduct of the same inflammatory processes that occur in the arterial wall.

While medically this is very debatable, clinically both heart disease and dementia patients have similar lifestyles. In my experience, cleaning up the lifestyle of anyone with CNS symptoms greatly enhances their quality of life.

An alkaline diet, moderate exercise of an hour per day, and nutraceuticals that address inflammatory pathways combined with meditative or relaxation therapy work better than any known drug for our clients. Hundreds of physicians that practise anti-aging medicine report that "medicine is great at the treatment of acute illness, and horrible for chronic debilitating conditions."

Dr. David Purelmutter, a practising neurologist in Florida, attacks the inflammatory processes of the modern world in his patients with a host of natural and medical alternatives. His results are nothing less than astounding. With gluten-free diets, hyperbaric oxygen, intravenous vitamins, minerals, and antioxidants, rehabilitative exercise programs, and a sincere desire to give back quality of life to his patients, his work adds to the options of what is now possible for patients with neurological diseases.

I recommend that everyone read his books: *Grain Brain, The Better Brain Book*, and also his book on children's early brain development. Happy healthy people who eat great food and exercise often age exceptionally well compared to the average population, in my experience.

You've Learned a New Language

The information in this book is highly detailed and you have stayed with reading it thus far. You have discovered that it is no longer remotely possible to trust our food supply or the health care system you live in. Every person must consciously take responsibility for themselves and their loved ones, and boldly go back to where our ancestors were. Taking responsibility for your carbohydrate metabolism, fat intake, and quality of foods by eating organic food and high-quality fat and protein. These terms now must become part of your common vocabulary about the life you live.

Like any new language, once you become familiar and conversant, it becomes second nature. The conversation we have begun with our personal interactions between food, lifestyle, and environment now affords the added benefit of reducing real risk and increasing quality of life. My own life and research with patients has proven this is NOT speculation, and that these tools yield a longer and a higher quality of life.

A Tibetan Lama said to me once, *"Everything I have told you I would expect you to be suspicious of. Please go out into your world and put it to the test and prove me wrong."* I offer the same challenge to you. *Live the lifestyle and see if you are gaining benefit.*

With Stark simplicity, you must now practice the methods with which to live a more vibrant and risk-free life. Embed them into the very core of your existence by rote memory. Become proactive, seeking out high-quality sources of food, exercise, entertainment, and relaxation in your life. It is hard work, but will bring richer rewards than you might begin to imagine.

Take the Rocking Chair Test and Get Motivated!

The motivational coach, Anthony Robbins, gives the analogy of a rocking chair test. He suggests that you first imagine yourself sitting in a rocking chair. It's at the end of your life. You're looking back over all of the things that you've done. How would you feel if you did or did not participate in an activity in your life many years before when you had the chance?

In my particular situation, I imagine a life without ever having flown my paraglider, never being able to fly 3000 feet above a French village, eye-to-eye with a hawk. It would be a life where I never circled above a pristine lake in the Rocky Mountains with two bald eagles on my wing. It would be a life of never being able to take my friends and loved ones with me on my tandem paraglider and broadening their vistas, sharing our adventures. A life without this would be inconceivable. And so, having regret and remorse over not doing these things in my life, the thought became the impetus for taking action to become a pilot and get my feet off the ground. The same test was used for the writing of this book and the others to come also. I have a message to give, I must honor it and get off my butt and do it. Stay motivated and focused and enjoy what life will bring you when you stay consistent – on course, and with excellent lifestyle habits to support you!

Now this rocking chair test must be used with the basic things in life, like the way you eat, exercise, handle stress, and lastly, enjoy your life. The "cost and benefit" of your lifestyle must be considered.

It seems very simple to me to look at the way I eat and see the effect over time of doing it correctly and what would happen if I did it incorrectly. This motivates me to get it right most of the time. What does it take to motivate you to get it right most of the time? Dying a slow death of cancer is a reality for three out of seven individuals. Likewise, one out of two women will die of heart disease. How much pain and suffering will it take for you to understand *you have a choice with every bite, with every plate, and with every few hours that you have to renew yourself* with food?

Exercise is a Powerful Mood Elevator

It seems very simple to look at the way one exercises to see the effect over time. Basic moderate exercises on a daily basis are a necessity. Exercise increases lean muscle mass, decreases body fat, and improves cardiovascular and aerobic condition. Did you know that exercise is the number-one mood-elevating drug? Not exercising is the antithesis of all these benefits.

Sit back in your rocking chair, and look at the next 5, 10, and 20 years and see what your life would be like without exercise. Now try to imagine 5 years of fairly consistent exercise and the benefits you would gain. Being the mood-elevating drug, I can almost guarantee you unimaginable gain in your personal life in almost every facet.

It seems very simple to look at the way one thinks and see its effects over time. Negativity, hate, anger, frustration, and fear all have negative effects on the vitality of the brain, organ function, and immune system. Becoming aware of these emotions makes it easy to choose not to participate with them. Yes, every day these emotions may come up, but you have to do all that is within your power to let go of them, by taking positive actions to resolve issues that create negative emotions.

Correspondingly, optimism, love, joy, and courage have very positive effects on the human body. Over a period of time – 10 or 20 years – you can visually see how someone wears his or her emotional state on the physical body.

Sit back in your rocking chair and imagine a life with both mental constructs and feel deep down in your bones how it would be to live one way and the other, then place that picture in your mind every morning before you get out of bed. Motivation is most effective from the inside out!

The Illusion That Food is all You Need to Survive Can Take up to 30 Years off Your Life Span

It seems very simple to look at the way I eat, the foods to select from, and the fact that I will need to take a handful of vitamins daily for the rest of my life. High on a sacred peak, there's a little sunny plot of land with vegetables and fruits tended lovingly by monks who chant holy words, but I have yet to find their local outlet or retailer. Walking into the market, seeing foods that have been transported, fumigated, chilled, wrapped, and radiated – all possibly up to four weeks prior – leaves me with little doubt for the need of a little insurance.

The supplementation of nutrients to our diet will help all of us maintain a balance more easily in our modern world. Nutraceuticals that mimic nature in their concentrations, preparations, and cleanliness are the only way to assure that biological pathways have the ammunition to fight the battles our environment brings us. Adding ionized alkaline water technology can also give advantage to the basics of life. Wanting to live a longer life means I have to use tools that work in my world. On a day-to-day basis, I feel better taking my supplements and you now can make the same informed choices.

It seems possible to me that every successive decade, my mental and physical performance seem unchangeable. The truth is, I don't see myself sitting in a rocking chair. I see myself making rocking chairs and one day just closing up the workshop and taking a walk, never to return. This may be a dream, but it is the dream I choose to live, and so far, it's working. You, too, can choose any dream you wish to live.

Using the tools of lifestyle, with all the facets shining like a splendid diamond in the sunlight, work to keep the stone polished. It's hard work in this life, and yet we must maintain dignity without bowing down to inferior foods, thoughts, activities, or lack of control over our free will. *And by our actions, so shall we be.* There is such inspiration in this beautiful world, and we need to choose it carefully. Only by doing this, do we collect enough personal power to significantly help others. The proper use of this power ends suffering, not only of ourselves, but also to our families first, our villages second, and lastly, our world. The work is straightforward and is moment-by-moment.

What we choose to do in each and every day rewards us without prejudice. Destiny? I rightly think the sum total of our actions is destiny. You have the tools to make your health and heart destiny now. What will motivate you to live without mental or physical pain? What will get you out exercising on a regular basis? What will inspire you to cook and plan great meals at home?

It seems STARK simple: LIVE NOW, DIE LATER!

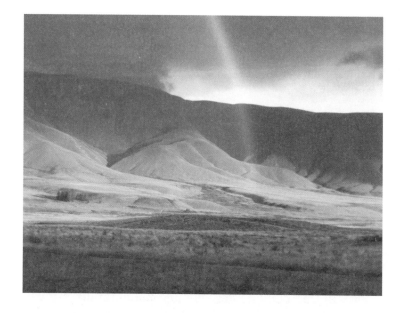

LIVE NOW – DIE LATER

PART FOUR

THE STARK HEALTH DIET AND LIFESTYLE

CHAPTER NINETEEN
Getting It All Together

What constitutes our lifestyle is molded by many factors: social convention, peer pressure, habit, or believing you are doing the right thing. People do not achieve the results they want because they never have clearly defined their health and performance intentions.

So, in this particular section, it's important that you clearly define your intentions. If you picked up this book, your intentions are somewhat similar to mine. You most likely want to "live now," with a very high quality of life and "die later" with very little pain and very little downtime! If this seems like an admirable existence and goal, then I expect you to quit unfruitful activities and join me in a STARKHEALTHY life-style!

Every time you eat, drink, exercise, rest, and fortify your body, you make a choice. I will provide you with the simple rules that I have proven to work – first with myself in my dire health situation and secondly, with my patients. These incalculable assets are gained from the wisdom that comes from experience. Wisdom is the practice of learning from your mistakes and observations and applying that knowledge the next time. For example, my father had only an 8th-grade education, yet he became one of the best thoroughbred trainers and breeders in the United States because of his powers of observation. He was able to take horses that others would discard as being broken or over the hill and rebuild them into champions. His desire for me was to be a veterinarian, and in as much taught me the rules of animal medicine as he saw them.

"Animals need very few things to be healthy and fulfill their potential – clean water, clean food, sunlight, regular exercise, and undisturbed

sleep, " he would tell me. "Add a little time and understanding and you can fix most things, " he said. I never made it to veterinary school, but after 35 years I can stand here and say that my father was right.

The enormity and complexity of the issues talked about in this book can be left behind. You don't need to remember all the mechanisms of how a person develops diabetes, heart disease, high cholesterol levels, blood clots, osteoporosis, cancer, and dementia. But you do have to remember the things that you must do to create results of your intentions. You will be amazed at just how short and complete these answers to the game of life really are.

Using these tools on a daily basis will allow you to have a personal freedom and clarity in the area of your health and life that you may never have had before. You will know from personal experience that your life-style is giving you a foundation of health, vitality, and spirit unattainable by any other means.

There's another thing you should know. When you use all the tools together, a synergistic effect occurs that begins to create incredible personal power. *This confidence is not a panacea – it comes via experience!* It is no guarantee that you will not be struck down by one of the inequities of living in a modern world. However, my experience and research have together given me unshakable confidence that between 60 and 80 percent of the risks which "common" people are exposed to can be eliminated. There are no drugs that can do this for you – you must do them for yourself. Mark Wayne Anderson, MD, states, "5 percent of the people who are sick consume 50 percent of the medical resources, the rest 'not sick' consume the remaining 48 percent and the exceptionally healthy lifestyle people 2 percent of the resources." Yes, we can change our health destiny and be the healthy 2 percent!

Your inspiration for life and living will come from unique areas. These should help you clarify your intentions. Then with these most effective mechanisms in place, you will be able to reap the benefits of a long and vital life. The best time to begin this type of work is prior to conception! If you are fortunate to have the one out of one million parents who did some of this work for you, then congratulations! You have been given a wonderful gift that blesses you throughout life. The rest of us can begin with the first tool by using the primary element of Chinese medicine – water.

CHAPTER TWENTY
So Vital and So Important

Doctors are trained about water and the human body in terms of crisis intervention. Electrolyte disturbances and dehydration are the primary concerns. Beyond that, the subtleties of the human body and its requirements for proper hydration are not really emphasized in the medical curriculum. In my search for the primary elements of health, water was grossly underrepresented.

Most public health officials talk about contamination to the water supplies from bacteria and parasites. They report on heavy metal toxicity of drinking water and issues that result from industrial chemical contaminants. Better filtration of the water and the process of chemically altering the water to kill bacteria have been straightforward approaches to water safety and health. Medically, we now can conclude that chronic dehydration and chronic illness may be underlying circumstances which the vast majority of the population is predisposed to.

What the French Found Out About Water

The French began investigating the water in their country before the turn of the 19th century. Their inquiry was pragmatic; they wanted to know if there were specific types of water that helped people live longer, more vibrant lives. As you would expect, they did find some correlation. Water, which came from underground artesian systems, was heavily laden with minerals and this appeared to help people live better.

When everything in the lifestyle appears to be the same, and the only difference is the water source and those people who drink a certain type of water found in one location demonstrate a marked longevity, you have to ask the question, what's in the water? The "Fountain of Youth" is the mythological bubbling spring, which gives eternal youth when one drinks it! Kings throughout history have sent forth adventurers looking for this elusive prize. To the best of my knowledge, they all came home empty-handed.

Japanese Discoveries from Water Research

What I did find, was a group of Japanese scientists who asked the question: If there are unique areas on the planet in which people appear to live longer and more vibrantly than in other areas, does the quality or characteristics of their water supply have any bearing on longevity? Do the water supplies between these populations have any similarities in the laboratory?

Yes was the answer. After quantifying the assays of water from different regions around the planet, it surprised them to find that the similarities were unmistakable. All the life-giving waters were saturated with calcium, magnesium, and potassium. Additionally, the waters were generally slightly to very alkaline in nature. Their pH was 7.0-10. Next and even more exciting was that the electrical properties of the water had a certain oxidation-reduction potential or ORP level.

The fresh water found in remote parts of the world was electrically charged negative, and thus able to pick up free radicals. *What this was saying to me was the water itself acted as an antioxidant!* It certainly coincided with current theories on the causes of aging and degeneration, thus explaining the long-lived populations who drank this water.

One additional property not expected, which demonstrated the uniqueness of fresh, alkaline, negatively ionized water, was the actual unique size of the cluster of water molecules when compared to regular water. The theory is, water molecules generally tend to join into clusters of between 11 to 15, making up a pretty large H20 molecule. The "special water" had clusters of 5 to 8 H20 molecules. This meant the water could actually hydrate more quickly, as it was physically "smaller," having less surface tension than regular water.

In summary the scientists concluded that the special water was electrically negative, with smaller clusters of molecules, highly dense with alkaline minerals and generally fresh out of the ground. Obviously the next question was how could scientists make water with similar properties in the laboratory?

Japanese Scientists Bring Their Findings to Millions

Through a complex system of electrolysis they were able to produce water that had almost identical properties to those found in remote regions of the Earth where people lived very healthy lives. Japan and Korea quickly went into the business of producing machines for home and hospital use that would produce ionized water. Today, while figures vary, it is estimated that about 20 percent of homes in Japan and Korea have one of these devices. My investigation further demonstrated much controversy about the efficacy and honesty of the industry that produces the water machines. Over the last couple of years I've been quietly going through the literature, looking at the arguments and while doing so, drinking lots of ionized water. I didn't want to miss out on an opportunity to create health.

The Research is Authenticated, Water is has a fourth phase !

As I mentioned before in the argument about osteoporosis, do you want to sitaround waiting for scientists to run studies on what works best and meanwhile watch your health worsen... or do you want to take action now and improve your health? Another example is multi-vitamins. As little as two years ago it was heresy to prescribe multi-vitamins to patients. Official policy suggested that our "diets are optimum and multi-vitamins are a waste of money." During the previous 50 years a groundswell of consumer activism went its own way. People did not need the blessings of their doctor any more. They felt healthier and lived better lives while taking multi-vitamins. Some estimates suggest almost 50 percent of the population was taking some form of multi-vitamin on a daily basis – against medical advice. I believe we are in a similar situation with ionized water.

I gave a lecture to a group of doctors in 2014 titled: "The Clinical Application of Energy Production, Oxygen State Physiology and Associated Cell and Mitochondrial Membrane Dynamics." As impressive as the title was, it took the newly discovered science of water and gave the doctors clinical relevance. Now they would know the science behind water and how to use it in their assessment and treatment of patients. Dr. Gerald H. Pollack, PhD, is the head of the Physical Chemistry Department at the University of Washington. He published a lifetime of work in late 2013 on the chemistry of water, something so fundamental you would have thought it was done decades earlier, however with new technology, he was able to state the following: *"Water has three phases – gas, liquid, and solid; but recent findings from our laboratory imply the presence of a surprisingly extensive fourth phase that occurs at interfaces. This finding may have unexpectedly profound implication for chemistry, physics and biology."*

When I read his book four times... It was clinically apparent, he had solved the mystery of water and how to use it. First, the ionization of water may in fact help to "structure water" for a more beneficial biological integration. Secondly, "structured water exists in every living plant and animal on the planet. When you eat a raw vegetable or fruit – the water in that food is immediately used in your body. It is 'an ungraded from of water.'" Your body would over time take ordinary tap water and "structure it" into H302, a negatively charged hexagram of six water molecules.

The Fountain of Youth

When not enough water is available, this structured water, which covers every membrane in all living tissue, has two ways to break down, which explains why chronic dehydration is chronic disease. In the presence of free water, the breakdown of "structured" water yields a couple of extra water (H_2O) molecules to be used later. However, when no "free water" is to be found, the breakdown of structured water yields super-oxide free radicals (O_2) and hydrogen peroxide (H_2O_2), which, as you might expect, are free radicals that can damage or accelerate cell biological systems' decline, tissue decline, and ultimately organ function. This is the basis for chronic disease from yet another vector. We are saying the live water from living plants or a quality ionizing machine is the fountain of youth!

My conclusion is, we should mimic the best water sources in the world, which have been proven by time and provided by technology. We should have in our homes "Stark-water" with the following properties: super hydrating, structured, appropriately alkaline mineral-laden, and electrically negative free-radical quenching water. To do this you first need a blender to increase your "live water" intake from fruits and vegetables, and then drink quality water each day as well.

What Not to Drink

When you compare standard water sources to the structured water properties just described, this is what is found:

1. From a purely environmental point of view, 15 billion plastic water bottles per year are being placed into landfills. Having your own machine completely eliminates your personal part in this environmental problem. Having a blended drink in a thermos fortifies your body too.

2. Most bottled water and energy drinks used for fluid replacement are very acidic in nature, and some of them are as low as 3.5 on the pH scale. They can contain colorings known to cause mood disturbances and multiple other symptoms. The high phosphate content of carbonated drinks greatly contributes to loss of calcium from bone, metabolic processes, and fluid balance. NFKB is also increased with chronic acid dietary intake leading, to a greater chance of uncontrolled tumor growth.

3. The ORP of tap water and bottled water is positive, while ionized water is negative. Water with a positive ORP becomes a source of free radicals, as we have seen.

4. A glass of freshly blended carrots and apples can have enough free radical-quenching power to have a negative charge of −200 millivolts (mv).

5. When the ORP of the waters of our isolated and pure places was tested, some of them came to over −400 mv. Machine water with new technology has reached −800 mv. Generally speaking, acidic water and manufactured liquids are creating oxidative damage with their positive ORP levels. Stay away from them or die early in my opinion.

6. Tap water and spring water generally are the best choices if you do not have access to an Alkaline Ionizing machine. Distilled and "pure water" can actually upset mineral

balance in the body in addition to not having any minerals at all.

7. As most commercial water products and soft drinks are acidic – this includes the homemade carbonated drinks – acidity kills the "living" water; the mineral balance is not good for animals either. Going back to my father's knowledge, I recall him telling me, "You cannot raise good stock unless you have hard water." He knew, as do farmers all over the world, that calcium, magnesium, and potassium are the alkaline macro-minerals vital for health.

Why Drink Water? What Are the Benefits?

You will notice that when you drink structured water, it tastes smoother, does not fill you up, quenches your thirst, and actually makes you crave more water. Additionally, you may notice that you are sleeping better, thinking more clearly for longer periods of time, and have better resistance to colds and the flu. I have noticed many of these things myself. When you drink water of this quality, it immediately gets absorbed into your blood system and lymphatic system. This is good and facilitates the detoxification of all cells in your body, and at the same time, it allows quicker and more efficient nutrient delivery to each and every cell. Your lymphatic system is a major system of the body that is responsible for immunity. This system disposes of waste products whilst helping immune system cells move to their target locations to do their work.

How Much Water Should You Drink?

For most people, the answer will be between 2 and 3 liters / quarts per day. The best way to do this is to immediately drink a full 1 to 2 glasses of water first thing in the morning. Do this before you do anything else. Next, up to 30 minutes before and 30 minutes after meals, drink one-half glass. In between meals, drink an additional 1 to 2 glasses of water. Finally, before you go to bed drink 1 to 2 glasses of water.

Of course, you will have to get up and urinate and this will be a nuisance for anywhere from 4 to 6 weeks for most people. After that, your body will get used to this amount of fluid and you will find it "normal for you" as you go about your daily business. You will also find it difficult to drink anything but ionized water, as the costs to your health when going without will become readily apparent.

Lastly, the "official" guidelines are to drink half of your body weight in ounces. For example, if you weigh 180 pounds, drink a total of 90 ounces of water per day. Other recommendations say 1 milliliter per calorie consumed, so a 2000-calorie diet would require 2000 ml or 2 liters of water to be drunk during the day.

A very interesting fact I have noticed with my patients who drink ionized water is that they seem to have better kidney function. Creatinine levels are a standard medical test for kidney function because it has a very predictable rate of excretion. We can use the circulating amount of creatinine in the blood to calculate the efficiency of the kidneys.

In general terms, the average middle-aged person in my practice will have a kidney function between 65 to 75 percent; this is called the estimated "GFR." The person who has been drinking ionized water seems to have kidney function between 85 to 120 percent. This is quite startling as kidney function generally declines by 1 percent per year for the general population past the age of 40. Does drinking this water make your kidneys 20 years younger? According to my testing so far, I see a trend. This is a good thing. The Chinese experts who have studied this carefully for 2000 years report that one should drink enough water to urinate five long voids per day, in my experience you will have about 30 percent greater fluid intake than usual recommendations.

Closer to 3 liters is the guideline for most people if you take ancient advice from the experts. This always depends on your personal weight. When I was in medical school we learned in Physiology that the body can use about a liter of water per hour and loses water through the skin as sweat, the kidneys as urine, and the lungs as water vapor. Think of "steamy windows" as teenagers and you can see how much water gets blown away.

Thus the last rule would be to keep a glass by the bed and if you do get up in the middle of the night drink a half glass of water also. This last suggestion is Ayurvedic wisdom and predates Chinese medicine by 3000 years.

Water Ionizers and Blenders in the Home or Office?

If you have the ability to purchase a water ionizer, I would recommend it. A blender on the other hand is a kitchen appliance. In my book it's refrigerator, stove, blender. And as with ionizers, there are many brands available. Find a company that has been around a while and has the following.

When choosing blenders or ionizers for the home, look for these three features:

1. A 5-year-to-life warranty from the manufacturer is common in the better machines and gives peace of mind. Some have lifetime warranties!

2. Self-cleaning electrics that do not turn the machine off for any period of time for ionizers and easy cleaning for blenders.

3. Ionizers that can produce at least 3 liters per minute of ionized water and ones that can maintain an ORP reading of –250 or greater.

Expect to invest $500 to $3500 US for a machine depending on the quality. The pay back time is usually under two years if you think about how much less of a consumer you will be of "convenience foods" and water. You will turn the page on eating out less because your easy to make and tasty smoothies are energizing and the correct amount of water on board turns off the aberrant hunger reflexes created by the additives in store bought food. Yes, they really do that to us...

Water is an essential element. It has a profound effect on every aspect of human performance from mental agility, physical coordination, illness prevention, and recovery. If you cannot get hold of a home ionizer, alkaline water, spring, artesian water, or tap water will be better than any other commercially available source. One two or three smoothies per day also will really change your life too.

The technology of structured alkaline water has improved upon what most municipal water supplies offer and eliminates the uncertainty about purity and the pollution associated with plastics. After my exploration into the field of water and health, it would appear to me this quoted line is true most of the time: "You're Not Sick–You're Thirsty!" (K. Batamanghelidj, M.D., noted author and hydration researcher).

CHAPTER TWENTY-ONE
Your Food Is Your Lifeline

Processed, sterilized, packaged, then cleverly marketed, our modern food supply has created the epidemic problem of inflammation and early decay which is what the majority of us are suffering from.

Eating right will change the way your body uses its number-two drug, which is FOOD! The STARKHEALTH rules are simple and the types of food you can eat are sustainable and healthy. However, you must have enough personal power to say, "I am worth the effort necessary to make my food choices with care and reverence." Once you do this, you can succeed like so many others have.

Many people want to see a diet in a format that describes what to eat and what not to eat. Although I have done this in words, it's often easier to see it in a list or other format whereby a quick glance will help cement it into the memory banks. This chapter is for that purpose.

First, you'll see a diagram that "illustrates the WHY" to follow this STARKHEALTH plan. The diet will follow.

Dietary Pathogenesis: How our health declines from the foods we eat.

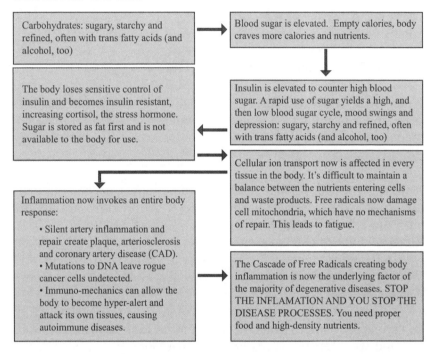

Carbohydrates: sugary, starchy and refined, often with trans fatty acids (and alcohol, too)

Blood sugar is elevated. Empty calories, body craves more calories and nutrients.

The body loses sensitive control of insulin and becomes insulin resistant, increasing cortisol, the stress hormone. Sugar is stored as fat first and is not available to the body for use.

Insulin is elevated to counter high blood sugar. A rapid use of sugar yields a high, and then low blood sugar cycle, mood swings and depression: sugary, starchy and refined, often with trans fatty acids (and alcohol, too)

Cellular ion transport now is affected in every tissue in the body. It's difficult to maintain a balance between the nutrients entering cells and waste products. Free radicals now damage cell mitochondria, which have no mechanisms of repair. This leads to fatigue.

Inflammation now invokes an entire body response:

- Silent artery inflammation and repair create plaque, arteriosclerosis and coronary artery disease (CAD).
- Mutations to DNA leave rogue cancer cells undetected.
- Immuno-mechanics can allow the body to become hyper-alert and attack its own tissues, causing autoimmune diseases.

The Cascade of Free Radicals creating body inflammation is now the underlying factor of the majority of degenerative diseases. STOP THE INFLAMATION AND YOU STOP THE DISEASE PROCESSES. You need proper food and high-density nutrients.

Established Scientific Position on Dietary Effects on the Degenerative Diseases of Heart Disease, Cancer, and Diabetes

What do the foremost-researched scientists and governing bodies have to say about the specific connection between primary degenerative disease and diet? Remember, these people are usually very conservative in their recommendations.

The American Heart Association

"A healthy diet and lifestyle are your best weapons to fight cardiovascular disease. Remember, it's the overall pattern of your choices that counts."

The American Cancer Society

- *"Eat a healthy diet, with an emphasis on plant sources.*

- *Choose foods and drinks in amounts that help achieve and maintain a healthy weight.*

- *Eat 8 or more servings of a variety of vegetables and fruits each day.*

- *Choose whole grains over processed (refined) grains.*

- *Limit intake of processed and red meats.*

- *Drink no more than 1 drink per day for women or 2 per day for men."*

New Zealand Ministry of Health - Food and Nutrition Guide-lines for Healthy Adults: Diabetes

"The aim of dietary intervention is to improve all the biochemical and physiological parameters associated with Type 2 Diabetes. The maintenance of blood glucose levels alone will help prevent the micro-vascular complications of diabetes. Because most people die from the cardiovascular complications associated with diabetes, dietary advice to lose weight, reduce blood pressure and improve lipid profiles (including HDL and triglycerides) is important.

In addition, reduced intake of total fat, particularly saturated fat, (I don't agree with this statement as its based on an unproven medical bias – stay away from vegetable fats with the exception of extra virgin olive oil) may reduce the risk for diabetes. Increased diabetes incidence is reported with increased intake of dietary fat, independent of total energy (American Diabetes Association 2003). It appears that all types of dietary fat (except omega-3 fatty acids) may have an adverse effect on insulin sensitivity. Other studies have shown a reduced risk with increased intake of whole grains and dietary fiber (American Diabetes Association 2003). Although moderate alcohol intake has been related to improved insulin sensitivity, there is insufficient data to support a specific recommendation for moderate alcohol intake to reduce the risk in developing Type 2 Diabetes (American Diabetes Association 2003)."

While I consider myself to be *"conservatively radical"* compared to mainstream medical opinion, the most medically prudent associations and consumer advocates have all come in agreement with the side of reason that says, EAT YOUR VEGGIES AND FRUIT WITH VERY LITTLE RED MEAT!

Also, they agree that by not eating right, you will without a doubt become part of the statistics of one of the three major causes of modern death: CAD, Cancer, and Diabetes.

Diabetes and the Glycemic Index of Foods

Robert Lustig, MD and pediatric endocrinologist at the University of San Francisco, makes two very poignant statements: "The average insulin level and glucose level have doubled in the last 20 years," and, "the fastest growing obese segment in the population is six months old to three years!"

It is obvious, if we take a stab at stopping all three deadly diseases in their tracks, we must start with diabetes and blood sugar control. By gaining blood sugar control, we reduce our overall risk very significantly. As the New Zealand guidelines point out, "A low glycemic diet combined with low fat intake will greatly improve insulin sensitivity and reduce diabetes risk." Becoming an expert on glycemic index and glycemic load is a lot easier than getting a drivers license. Learn it, master it, and use it for life. Go straight to the source online. In my experience, this is the best way to have a good overview of the topic.

Resource: www.glycemicindex.com

STARKHEALTH DIETARY SUGGESTIONS

THE "STARK DIET" is as easy as 1-2-3. The Stark Diet is by default, a diet that has a low glycemic load. For further information refer to University of Sydney's GI website in addition to www.glycemicindex.com. Sticking to the "5-4-3-2-1" axiom will leave you in the best possible position to fight aging and increase vitality each and every day.

The 5-4-3-2-1 STARK-SIMPLE Plan is listed below. It's easy; just spend two minutes reading over it and you'll see why I say it's easy.

The 5-4-3-2-1 STARK-SIMPLE Plan:

5 big servings of fresh non-starchy veggies per day (50 percent raw)

4 servings of fresh fruits per day leaving out bananas, figs and dried fruits (50 percent raw)

3 servings (60 gm,s or 2.5 oz) of lean protein (wild fish, nuts, wild meat, and free range everything else, in that order)

2 litres of (ionized if you can) water or enough to promote five very long urinations per day. 2 Green Veggie smoothies per day.

1 hour of exercise to stimulate the lymphatic and digestive systems, increase muscle tone, lower blood sugar, and increase insulin sensitivity.

1 serving of grain per day. This is a grain that is never processed, always fresh and wholesome. NEVER use gluten containing foods or corn products; they are the most hybrid of grains. Hybrid grains are genetically altered for modern farming needs – not nutritional content optimization.

If you stick to this formula in eating and exercise, most people will reduce body fat, increase lean muscle mass, have much more energy, sleep more soundly, and have a better overall disposition or mood. Diseases tend to reduce in occurrence by about 40 percent, and the quality of life is enhanced as well.

What about the Side Effects?

As "side effects" go, let's see if you can live with this one: anti-aging authors report 13 to 15 years of life expectancy increase!

CHAPTER TWENTY-TWO

Nutraceuticals - Special Vitamins, Specific to Your Body

It seemed obvious after 35 years of investigation, experimentation, and observation of my patients that vitamins were a foregone conclusion. That was not to be the case as the pharmaceutical industry, in collusion with standard medical practice, had been as efficient as a pest exterminator at creating doubt in the minds of the public about the use, safety, and validity of vitamins, while continuing a 20-year campaign to control and financially gain from the emerging industry.

Can Vitamins Harm?

Ask any street corner expert and you will get different and divergent views about the pros and cons of taking vitamins. "Vitamin A is toxic!" are words you will hear; yet in my career, I have never seen that happen or met another doctor who has either.

"Vitamin C in too high a dose causes kidney stones" are also words you will hear. And again, I have never met anyone that this has happened to, or seen one scientific paper that backs up the claim. On and on it goes, so you need the tools to know what is the state of this art and science and what benefit it will be to you? Will it help you to have a better quality of life for the sake of putting off the inevitable; in other words, if you take vitamins, will it have anything to do with helping you achieve the goal of "Live Now - Die Later"? My experience personally and professionally is YES! In 35 years of clinical experience, I can say, "a week does not pass without some form of miracle seen in my patients who were stymied by conventional medical care."

Synergistic Combinations Are Most Effective

I would like to share with you a small but important point when taking vitamin supplements. Taking single vitamins such as vitamin E, B, or C may actually create imbalances and especially when taken in high dosages for prolonged periods of time. It is interesting to note that you do not find problems when vitamin preparations are taken in combinations of 10 or more separate nutrients together.

As a doctor who prescribes very strong vitamins, it is important to know what formulations are best for what. For example, our basic multivitamins used in the clinic have more than fifty ingredients. All products that are combined together in the vitamin have been produced below body temperature, so as not to break down any of the naturally occurring enzymes found in pure, undisturbed natural form. After 35 years, I can say, "I have never seen a vitamin overdose." The prescriptive use of these "orthomolecular nutritional supplements" has been a specialty of chiropractic physicians since vitamins were first being made in Wisconsin in the 1920s by contemporaries of Dr. Price. These are "food supplements" first, and not drugs.

Jonathan Wright, M.D., is the father of bio-identical hormone replacement therapy. This is now the cornerstone of anti-aging medicine; he eloquently cautions that we do not know how an individual's body uses vitamins, minerals, and antioxidants until we measure exactly what goes in and what comes out via various pathways. One person may have an extremely efficient metabolic elimination of hormone by-products or vitamin by-products, while the next person may retain very high levels within their system.

Giving two people the same dosage based on body weight would likely present entirely different results in a clinical setting, as one person may have too much hormone or vitamin on board while the next person may not have enough retained to have an effect. And yes, this goes for pharmacy prescriptions, too. This is why our extensive blood tests are used to lead us toward better outcomes when prescribing nutraceuticals.

When we do a large array of laboratory tests, which include inflammation markers, multiple hormone systems, electrolyte levels, and immune system competency, we can begin to get a look at patients' individual requirements. Keying out disease processes is relatively easy compared to forecasting degenerative pathways based on early trends. Physicians such as Dr. Wright and myself are hopeful the rest of our fraternity will see this as the most effective place to begin healthcare – before the pathology develops.

Over the course of time, clinicians, myself included, who have formulated synergistic vitamin supplements for specific reasons such as fatigue, depression, repair, and immune system support, have found a "middle line" that is effective for most and simply regulating the dosage up or down achieves great clinical responses. Contrast this to walking into your pharmacy and picking up a "one per day" multi-vitamin and mineral supplement. You can count on the fact they will be synthetic, as that is the cheapest method of production, and secondarily the formulation will be minimal. Synthetic vitamins can block natural vitamin synthesis and have been linked to increasing certain diseases such as lung cancer, for instance synthetic beta-carotene.

What Does the Research Say About Multi-vitamins?

The following definitive study on multi-vitamins clearly points out just how little research has been done in this area. The term "poorly nourished" is well-chosen and demonstrates how easily scientific literature can mislead the majority of clinicians. We assume that the "poorly nourished patient" would be of lower social economic status, poorly educated, and easily identified by "the system" as having a high probability of poor nutritional status. Nothing could be farther from the truth; over 90 percent of the general population is, in fact, "poorly nourished." I may add that the increased consumption of carbohydrates in the diet created by food cravings will accentuate a poorly nourished person's risk of developing degenerative disease.

Results? Few trials have addressed the efficacy of multi-vitamin/mineral supplement use in chronic disease prevention in the general population of the United States. One trial on poorly nourished Chinese showed supplementation with combined beta-carotene. vitamin E. and selenium reduced gastric cancer incidence and mortality, and overall cancer mortality.

In a French trial, combined vitamin C, vitamin E, beta-carotene, selenium, and zinc reduced cancer risk in men but not in women. No cardiovascular benefit was evident in both trials. Multi-vitamin/mineral supplement use had no benefit for preventing cataracts. Zinc/ antioxidants had benefits for preventing advanced age-related macular degeneration in persons at high risk for the disease.

With few exceptions, neither beta-carotene nor vitamin E had benefits for preventing cancer, cardiovascular disease, cataracts, and age-related macular degeneration. Beta-carotene supplementation increased lung cancer risk in smokers and persons exposed to asbestos (this was synthetic beta-carotene). Folic acid alone or combined with vitamin B12 and/or vitamin B6 had no significant effects on cognitive function. Selenium may confer benefits for cancer prevention but not cardiovascular disease prevention. Calcium may prevent bone mineral density loss in post-menopausal women, and may reduce vertebral fractures, but not non-vertebral fractures.

The evidence suggests dose-dependent benefits of vitamin D with/ without calcium for retaining bone mineral density and preventing hip fracture, non-vertebral fracture, and falls. We found no consistent pattern of increased adverse effects of multivitamin/mineral supplements except for skin yellowing by beta-carotene.

Conclusion. Multi-vitamin/mineral supplement use may prevent cancer in individuals with poor or suboptimal nutritional status (THIS IS ABOUT 90 PERCENT OF THE POPULATION). The heterogeneity in the study populations limits generalization to United States populations. Multi-vitamin/mineral supplements conferred no benefit in preventing cardiovascular disease or cataracts, and may prevent advanced age-related macular degeneration only in high-risk individuals. The overall quality and quantity of the literature on the safety of the multi-vitamin/mineral supplements is limited.[1]

My Recommendation About Vitamins

We have to ask the question; why are their more people suffering from the diseases of obesity and its related chronicity's than malnutrition and starvation on the planet at this time? As you can gather from the above article, it's not a simple matter. What I have discovered over the course of my career is that synergy truly means what it implies – the whole is truly greater than the sum of its parts

[1] Huang HY, Caballero B, Chang S, Alberg A, Semba R, Schneyer C, Wilson RF, Cheng TY, Prokopowicz G, Barnes II GJ, Vassy J, Bass EB. Multivitamin/Mineral Supplements and Prevention of Chronic Disease. Evidence Report/ Technology Assessment No. 139. (Prepared by The Johns Hopkins University Evidence-based Practice Center under Contract No. 290-02-0018). AHRQ Publication No. 06-E012. Rockville, MD: Agency for Healthcare Research and Quality. May 2006.

as they act together, providing even greater than expected results. *First and foremost, the assimilation of nutrients must be done in an appropriate environment.* The digestive tract is everything, and maintaining proper digestive pH for the breakdown and absorption of fats, carbohydrates, and protein is essential. The Stark Diet ensures you have the right amount of soluble and insoluble fiber that will become a good home for digestive flora. After establishing this, high-quality fermented products such as pickles, onions, vinegars, yogurt, and other cultured foods will help keep your own internal compost pile working beautifully. It is in this environment that you can get maximal absorption of minerals, vitamins, and enzymes. The facts that agriculture is a for-profit business and that profit is based on weight and volume lead us to the conclusion that the nutritional component of the food being produced is secondary to its ability to generate profit. Disease resistance and portability are the most important factors in bringing a foodstuff to the market. Over the course of time, this "mono culture" has delivered to us – one crop at a time – record amounts of food. Warehouses, granaries, silos, and freezing facilities maintain the world supply of food. The balance that should occur from your fresh Stark Diet cannot occur due to the source of that diet.

The fact that agriculture is a for-profit business and that profit is based on weight and volume, not nutritional content. leads us to the conclusion that the nutritional component of the food being produced is secondary to its ability to generate profit, and health benefits are not considered.

Fresh food, multi-vitamins, minerals, and enzymes, in addition to antioxidants, are the smart person's best insurance in an uncertain world. We are all too often concerned about the catastrophic recovery from illness or injury devoting all of our attention and resources into systems that will keep us from financial and physical harm – namely necessary insurance coverage. Rarely do we find individuals that are proactive in taking care of themselves – to ensure higher fitness, performance, and immunity from disease. In fact, you were probably unaware that you had any control over this to any substantial degree before reading this book. So what are the minimal amounts of vitamins and minerals necessary to take to give us baseline insurance?

In my estimation, a minimal program that everyone should be on, regardless of age or sex, should include a multi-vitamin to compensate for farming practices, an antioxidant to further compensate for storage and delivery issues, a multi-mineral that can be included in the multi-vitamin to further guarantee the trace elements necessary to fuel metabolism, and lastly, something specifically to fight inflammation, such as fish oil. In my opinion, with these three or four products, many health issues which affect most of the population can be greatly reduced or eliminated.

How to Choose a Multi-Vitamin

As stated previously, my personal multi-vitamin has over 50 individual nutrients in its formulation. Its composition is:

- Vitamin A 2000 IU
- Vitamin D3 400 IU
- Vitamin E 200 IU
- Vitamin C 1000 mg
- Vitamin B6 25 mg
- Vitamin B1 13 mg
- Vitamin B2 10 mg
- Niacin 45 mg
- Vitamin B 12 30 mcg

- Pantothenic acid 50 mg
- Folic acid 200 mcg
- Biotin 400 mcg
- Calcium aspartate 101 mg
- Magnesium aspartate 100 mg
- Phosphorus chelate 20 mg
- Potassium proteinate 540 mcg
- Copper chelate 100 mcg
- Zinc aspartate 500 mcg
- Manganese aspartate 1.5 mg
- Molybdenum chelate 50 mcg
- Chromium chelate 25 mcg
- Selenium chelate 30 mcg
- Iodine 50 mcg
- Sodium proteinate 510 mcg
- Rubidium chelate 15 mcg
- Lithium chelate 0.8 mcg
- Lemon bioflavonoids 100 mg
- Rutin 25 mg
- Hesperidin complex 50 mg
- Choline bitartrate 100 mg
- Inositol 100 mg
- PABA 50 mg

- L-glycine 9.66 mg
- Chlorophyll 10 mg
- Vitamin F 5 mg
- L-phenylalanine 13 mg
- L-histidine 5 mg
- L-tyrosine 9 mg
- L-lysine 13 mg
- L-valine 15 mg
- dl-methionine 9 mg
- L-isoleucine 13 mg
- L-leucine 18 mg
- L-threonine 9 mg
- L-glutamic acid 2 mg
- Goldenseal root 45 mg
- Eleuthero root 45 mg
- Garlic bulb 40 mg
- Tillandsia 30 mg.

This is a supplement called "Core Level Health Reserve" by Nutri-West of Douglas, Wyoming.

As you can see, this is a complex formulation putting together vitamins, minerals, antioxidants, herbs, proteins, and amino acids that work synergistically. I have personally been taking this formula for 15 years now and consistently see enhanced well-being in myself and in patient populations of both mine and other doctors. *This is a prescription vitamin product administered under the care of an appropriately trained healthcare provider.*

From age five taking one half tablet per day up to a critically ill patient taking two tablets three times a day, this is a foundation product. Over-the-counter preparations found at health shops will rarely have this type of formulation. Vitamin D is essential, and the World Health Organization attributes over 30 percent of the 21 million cancers per year on the planet to lack of vitamin D. The above formula has 400 IU in it; however, you need more as you age because of decreased digestive ability to absorb it.[2]

In addition, very old people do not take the time to prepare high quality food for themselves and indirectly lose nutrients, such as protein, fat-soluble vitamins, and, of course, the active vitamins and enzymes of fresh food. Vitamin D should be in the "D3" form to be used effectively and 1200 to 3000 IU per day would be fine for anyone over the age of 15. (Dr. Mercola recommends 35 IU per pound of body weight; much higher than standard recommendations.)

The farther away you live from the equator (north or south), the greater your chances of being deficient. *"Gamers and IT people," who are notorious for avoiding the light of day, are at great risk of poor development to their bones, immune system, and general genetics.* These people should sun bathe or use tanning beds on a regular basis. Only 15 minutes of tanning bed three times per week in winter will keep most people who live in chilly climates out of danger in the winter. The amount of UVB you get is inversely proportional to the incidence of cancer![3] When the sun is high overhead, sit out and have a cup of green tea, a smoothie, or glass of

---

2 AEP Vol. 19, No. 7 Grant and Mohr July 2009: 446 - 454, 447

3 AEP Vol. 19, No. 7 Grant and Mohr July 2009: 446 – 454, 447

alkaline water for 10 to 15 minutes. That is tens of thousands of free vitamin D units!

Antioxidants

This word is as common as "corn starch," but what does it actually mean and why is it considered a priority in my lifestyle program? By definition, an antioxidant is a nutrient or chemical that reacts with and neutralizes free radicals or chemicals that release free radicals. Antioxidants are also called free radical scavengers. Vitamins A, C, E, and some of the B vitamins, beta-carotene, selenium, and some key enzymes in your body are all antioxidants.

However, the best source of these free radical scavengers is not taking a handful of vitamins and then eating what you want; it is having a control gate on the propagation of them in the first place, and then finding fresh natural sources of antioxidants, and lastly topping up with an array of tableted ones to ensure that the process is as good as possible. The science you have begun to understand in this book looks to fresh food that is grown as naturally as possible as the best source of nutrition, but consider the other side of the equation; everything we eat creates metabolic end products that produce free radicals. So how do you stop that, if free radical creation is part of the nutrient highway in the living metabolic processes?

Research into long-lived populations has shown that those who "under-eat" or have calorie-restricted diets seem to live longer. They are at the correct weight or underweight. They have a better power to weight ratio and seem to be of better physical stature than similarly aged people in the general population.

And lastly, they are mentally brighter for longer. My observation is simple. You see lots of overweight people in their 40s to 50s, not so many in their 70s and very few if any in their 90s. Why? Because they died of weight-related oxidative damage-generated diseases such as diabetes, heart disease, and cancer.

While "under-eating" is as popular as an atheist on the board of directors at the local church, it is a workable method of reducing free radicals in the body. This allows slower decline and longer life. It is the only proven method to actually prolong life in humans by an amazing 10 to 30 percent.[4] What would you do with those years? My suggestion is that by containing free radicals, keeping calories lower, concentrating antioxidants in the diet, the overall benefit would be longer life, fewer medical bills, and a more productive member of society.

Freshly picked fruits and veggies are best for phyto-nutrient levels of antioxidants. Ionized alkaline water in the diet will pick up free radicals, and lastly a broad based multi-vitamin, antioxidant formula would help. It is extremely important that the multi-vitamin is of the highest quality and "non-synthetic" in its manufacture. Do not get caught up thinking this "super-juice" or that "berry-concentrate" is all you need. Super foods are just that, super because of exceptional constellations of antioxidants, vitamins, minerals, and enzymes that make them aid the body's processes very effectively.

If you rate them on how powerful they are, you would have a list that looks like this: Acai berries from South America, the allium family (fresh garlic and onions), barley for its roughage and low glycemic properties, beans and lentils again as protein fiber and antioxidants, buckwheat, all green food, hot peppers are especially good for brain metabolism, all raw nuts and seeds with particular attention to brazil, almond, walnut, and pistachio, sprouts, and

---

[4] Willcox BJ, Willcox DC, Todoriki H, Fujiyoshi A, Yano K, He Q, Curb JD, Suzuki M. Caloric Restriction, the Traditional Okinawan Diet, and Healthy Aging: The Diet of the World's Longest-Lived People and Its Potential Impact on Morbidity and Life Span. Ann N Y Acad Sci. 2007 Nov;1114:434-55.

lastly fermented products like yogurt and kefirs. Not a donut or piece of toast in sight!

Additionally, what is obvious is the lack of animal products with the exception of yogurt. The best diet is a vegetarian diet; six days a week, it's Stark Simple. The foods above will give you energy and fill you up with fewer calories when you put them into the diet as a base. My suggestion to add rendered fish, fowl and beef stocks to soups as they add massive amounts of vitamins A, D, E, F and K which are the basis for immune system and bone health, not to mention balance of the bowel flora.

Your own body makes massive amounts of antioxidants, and it does this in synergy with bacteria in the gut. These friendly bacteria actually make high amounts of pantothenic acid that is crucial for fighting stress. Think of it as vitamins C's cousin. Of the 500 bacteria found in the trillions in the gut, vitamin K and biotin are essential to health. Those same bacteria also assist in breaking down carbohydrates that supply immediate energy needs in the bowel. Someone put a lot of work into designing a very comprehensive symbiotic system for humans.

Fish Oils as a Wonder Drug?

The actual acid nature of the average diet has effects on NF Kappa B and the body's ability to have inflammation at a cellular level. This long-term imbalance due to bad fats and sugars in the diet is the reason we need to have a powerful "anti-diet" food concentrate in our diet. Enter "fish oil" or specifically cold-water fish oil, which is distilled, filtered of all contaminants, and concentrated for its active ingredients of EPA and DHA (Omega 3 Fatty Acids). These fats turn off this metabolic shift and return the body to balance.

I think that in the modern world with food production the way it is, everyone should be taking about 2000 mg per day of good quality fish oil. The better the diet the less you have to take, however, those with symptomatic problems according to a conversation I had with Dr. Barry Sears, PhD., the Father of Fish Oil Research, says, "5,000-10,000 mg per day may be necessary for some people to shut down inflammatory pathways." Of course, anyone on medication needs guidance with this, especially if you're taking aspirin or other blood thinning compounds. The only type of fish oil we use in our clinic has never been exposed to oxygen. Oil likes to go rancid, so the fish are harvested and oil pressed out under a nitrogen-rich environment and directly sealed, never warming above body temperature and never seeing the light of day, which also can cause free radicals.

How Much Should You Take?: It Depends

Fish oils help all types of problems, as it is integral in the root cause of most issues of inflammation. If you have heart disease, 4 to 6 grams per day is recommended and the same would go for anyone with aches and pains; they are caused by inflammation... get it? Next, for persons with acute or chronic illness such as irritable bowel disease, multiple sclerosis, lupus, and rheumatoid arthritis, 6 to 10 grams may be necessary.

When you consume omega-3 fatty acids, it takes two to three weeks to chemically alter the pathways so you can see clinical benefits. So hang in there, natural vitamins, minerals, oils, enzymes, foods, and exercise all take time to work. Consistency is what you are looking for to make changes in the long-term function. By shutting down NFKB, you are reducing your chances of supporting illness. It's Stark Simple: if you don't clean the kitchen, you get rats! Pay careful attention to diet.

Under-Eat Prescription Drugs

Every major drug classification works to destroy symbiotic biological relationships, so only use them when absolutely necessary. Antibiotics kill your friends (good flora) while killing the bad guys too. Heart meds such as statins can kill muscle by destruction of the primary energy production unit in your cells – the mitochondria. Mood-elevating drugs alter normal feedback mechanisms in the brain making it difficult to control motor and autonomic nervous systems ("operation of heavy machinery or motor vehicles is not recommended"). So, "under-eating pharmacy drugs in your life is very good advice and, in my opinion, would trump caloric restriction for quality-of-life benefits, as we take far too many drugs!" (number 4 leading cause of death in US).

So What Am I Saying?

1. Take a multi-vitamin and mineral supplement twice per day, as there are water-soluble parts that will not last over four to eight hours before they wash out. If you're sick, take them three times per day to increase tissue levels.

2. Half of your diet should be made up of "Super Foods" and half your diet should be raw. Take an antioxidant supplement with a broad base and multiple vectors of plant sources of nutrients.

3. Take fish oils on a daily basis, minimum 2 grams, and more if you have problems.

4. If you have illness or are on prescription medication, see a specialist who uses therapeutic nutrition and get their advice. Specific products like resveratrol, CoQ10, and others are nice if you can afford them; however, the correct dosage and quality will be the most important questions to use them efficiently.

It's a Grey Area or a Rainbow, Depending on Where You're Sitting

Quality production of natural vitamin compounds is only done by a handful of companies. Sadly, many synthetically mass-manufactured vitamins are low-grade. Standardized, high-grade "nutraceuticals" are put together with the best technology with true freshness and preservation of quality. Things can be overlooked when working with abundant synthetics. A grey area exists in that these specialty products are too specific and powerful to be put on the supermarket shelf; yet doctors and health care practitioners who want the best for their patients want pharmaceutical quality and reproducibility from one batch to another.

The good news is healthcare practitioners have been using nutraceuticals for the last 50 years. Consistently improved formulations have an answer for most problems that affect us. I am my own case study, living proof that high-quality nutritional supplementation of antioxidants, vitamins, enzymes, and oils can help one overcome chemotherapy, cancer, and lassitude. But you must use the best and rely on the advice of someone who has knowledge in this field.

Why Such High Dosages?

In my experience, taking the recommended daily allowance is actually a good place to start, but clinically when someone has illness and you treat it using a vitamin, mineral, antioxidant, herbal, or enzyme preparation, you need more than you think to push the body back into balance again. We will use between 10 and 100 times the amount the body uses to saturate systems to get the desired results. This must be done with professional guidance, as combining too many medications just as providing too many vitamin supplements can have side effects. The good news is nutraceutical compounds rarely cripple and maim people.

Therapeutic Nutrition is Not the Practice of Medicine and They, "The Experts," Prove This to Us Daily

Experts are not as they seem. Mayo Clinic, one of the USA's premier and premium healthcare centers states on their website "CoQ10 does not have any large studies to support its claim for protection against the side effects of statin drugs." Imagine that! There's more. "No large studies have confirmed this theory, and current guidelines don't recommend routine use of Coenzyme Q10 in people taking statins." This statement was made by Dr. Thomas Behrenbeck, M.D., cardiologist at Mayo Clinic. In Canada, all prescriptions of statins are accompanied with CoQ10 supplementation. Why? The reduction of side effects from medication is the goal. You see, the socialized system costs less to run when you have fewer problems, so you learn to do it better, more efficiently and yes, help more people achieve fewer side effects. Now that's better medicine!

Why Would the Government Want to Protect You from Vitamins?

Many authors, including myself, have noticed that whenever the efficacy of vitamin compounds competes with something that can be a prescription product, government regulations are quick to come into place.

Vitamin B12 and folate are two examples where the dosage is regulated by government agencies so that doctors who have little training in nutrition can prescribe them at pharmacy rates. There are specific things to understand about disease states and these two vitamins, however, these two, along with a multitude of others, have been lobbied by the big pharmacy companies in the way that they become regulated, ultimately giving advantage to the big pharmacy companies. The loser in this regulated environment is you, the consumer, and oftentimes the alternative healthcare practitioner who cannot write prescriptions unless he is a medical doctor. Medical doctors who do write prescriptions for vitamin products are often scrutinized and singled out by their peers, as Dr. Sinatra will attest.

Chiropractors have always been the "alternative" to medical practice. In the USA, the training standards are equal to medical education. If there is a safe alternative to a pharmacy or surgical procedure, a chiropractor should know about it. Additionally, if a medical procedure or pharmacy would be more effective for the patient, the chiropractor is trained to refer in a timely manner. In my personal practice, I consistently refer patients for consultations with cardiologists, internists and general practitioners – it's just good for the patient.

How Do You Find Someone You Can Trust?

Good work stands out! Ask your friends, co-workers, and family if they've had an experience with practitioners that they felt really understood what the hell was going on. It must be someone who was clear, to the point, and effective in the situation they were consulted for. The American Academy of Anti-Aging Medicine will have a list of practitioners, but I caution that they will generally be medical doctors who will want to use bioidentical hormone therapy in addition to vitamins in their programs. Most will not have experience in using vitamins alone to engineer optimal health, let alone curing someone of let's say, irritable bowel syndrome. Chiropractors, naturopaths, herbalists, and acupuncturists may all be useful resources as are medical doctors trained in "functional medicine".

CHAPTER TWENTY-THREE

Laboratory Tests That Are Essential but Seldom Done Together

As a chiropractor and specialist in longevity medicine, my initial laboratory tests include over 60 separate assays. This is done to understand the function of the body as a "whole" system. You would think this would be common practice, however, it's rarely done. The difference between interventional medicine and preventative medicine really becomes clear when you look at laboratory testing. Do you think that laboratory test interpretation is "black and white"? Really it's not, and your health and future health depend on understanding what preventative medicine is all about.

When a laboratory does any particular test the doctor orders, it is returned to the doctor with a suggested "normal range." This is the heart of the issue – who sets these ranges? What is normal? What is optimal for each individual? That's the most important question! As a doctor, my reputation depends on my ability to discern normal from abnormal. For example, a middle-aged patient with a two-month history of fatigue, lassitude, and insomnia with a white blood cell count of 22,000 may have leukemia. The doctor would, of course, look at several other things, tests that would confirm the diagnosis, including a biopsy – but it's a pretty standard protocol. The normal level for the white blood cell count when I was in school was 5,000 to 9,000. Today, my local hospital tells me that the "normal range" is 4,500 to 11,000. This brings up the question of how this is determined and what it really means?

Seventy percent of the people who receive laboratory tests are in their last three years of life. Think about it, the older you get, the more likely it is you will become unwell and need to see the doctor. The other 30 percent who are being tested are those that doctors think may be sick and therefore, laboratory tests are performed. So, what should serve as a reference range for all is generally based on an old, ill population.

The interesting thing is, with very few exceptions, your doctor can't tell you the ideal levels that should be maintained throughout your life to keep you in top shape. The medical profession has never satisfactorily addressed concept of "optimal levels." Wouldn't it be good to have objective criteria that said your testosterone should be "X," your estrogen should be "Y"? What if you knew that you wanted your blood sugar at this level and your insulin at that? Further, what if you could say, "I can be relatively certain that if I keep these blood levels where they need to be, I will be far less likely to have diseases such as cancer, diabetes, and atherosclerosis"? The fact of the matter is, we do know what these optimal levels are! And if you do keep close to these levels, living to 90 to 100 years, still physically active, mentally sharp, and independent, can be a reality. This is the "Stark Reality" of what we are trying to get doctors and allied health care professionals to embrace.

Age Management's Effect on Mortality

The Cenegenics Health Institute in Las Vegas, Nevada, did a retrospective study of 4,000 patients who followed an anti-aging program for a period of five years. They cross-matched (compared) their patients who had been taking vitamins, bioidentical hormones, regular exercise, and stress reduction programs for five years, to 4,000 people of the same age in the general population. The results were startling.

For heart disease, America's number one killer at the time, over 12 percent of the general population between the ages of 40 to 74 years old had a heart attack. So, 480 or more cardiac events occurred in the general population group of 4,000. Half of these events, unfortunately, were fatal.

Remarkably, the patients that were following the health guidelines set out by the physicians at Cenegenics recorded only three cardiovascular events. That's right – 3 per 4,000 as opposed to 480 in 4,000! The conclusion, so eloquently put by Dr. Alan Mentz, was that "current trends in our patient population seem to be not doing any harm." (Yes, he may have suspected that he would be opening a can of worms, so he "understated" the elephant in the room.) Similar results were recorded for cancer, with 5,000 patients compared and only one case of cancer in the Cenegenics group, as opposed to over 600 for the general population.

The statistics for diabetes were equally impressive. In fact, not one new case of diabetes occurred in those following the anti-aging program during the five-year study.[5]

Is it All About Jobs?

You might think, and I would agree with you, that the medical world responded positively to this absolutely astonishing and revolutionary landmark study. No, they ignored it! There are really no drugs to sell as a consequence of this study or surgical procedures to perform. From my perspective, if you take that percentage of pathology out of the health care delivery system, it would not only

---

[5] IRB PROTOCOL Safety and Efficacy of Comprehensive Hormone Replacement, Low Glycemic Nutrition and Regular Exercise for Middle Aged Men and Women in a Community Setting, Alan Mentz, MD lecture of findings: 2003 AAFPRS Orlando, Fl. :Cenegenics Medical Institute in conjunction with the University of Tennessee.

destroy the established medical treatment protocol but the total investment in keeping the medical infrastructure as it is. This is anarchy and our results at Stark Health Centre back up the Cenegenics study.

What I Learned

I personally went through the Cenegenics program in Las Vegas as a doctor and patient. Over the course of my time there, it became apparent that desirable laboratory values were in the upper quartile of the normal range, or those equal to that of a healthy individual aged 25 to 35 years.

I happily discovered that my own levels, resulting from the program I had followed in the previous 15 years, were in the "zone." In fact, I recall Dr. Life (real name) asking me how much growth hormone I was taking when he reviewed my tests? I said to him that my research showed that hard physical exercise "to failure," specifically using leg muscles, would increase growth hormone as long as I continued to maintain a proper diet and sufficient sleep. He agreed that this was possible but had not seen it before.

The hierarchy of tests that I do and the way that I combine them are most logical. First and foremost, I tackle the big problem – heart disease. The following tests are the ones I've performed on every patient. You must also remember from our previous discussions that heart disease is an expression of silent inflammation, so it is important to check all inflammatory indicators.

* Please note – all tests are using European standard units and may be unfamiliar to Americans, the only country that uses that system of weight not volume, but that's another story.

CARDIAC LABORATORY TESTS

		UPPER 1/4	8.5.09	1/4	2/4	3/4	4/4
LABORATORY TEST	RANGE F/M	TARGET					
CARDIO							
hs-CRP	<3.0		1.43		1		
Homocysteine	5.0-15.0		5.2				1
Total Cholesterol	<4.0		4.2		1		
Trigs	<2.0		0.5				1
HDLs	>1.0		1.65			1	
LDLs	<2.0		2.3	1			
Trig/HDL ratio	<2.0		0.30				1
Fibrinogen	1.5-4.0		3.3		1		
CRR C/H	<3.5	2.5	2.5				1
Lipoprotein (a)	0-200		71				1
Insulin	10-80	<28	13				1
Vitamin D	50-150	>125	46*	1			
Urate or Uric Acid	0.14-0.37	<19.75	0.25		1		

I can see from this anonymous female patient's values that she's quite healthy. We did pick up that this 45-year-old aerobics instructor and organic gardener was not getting enough sun (deficient in Vitamin D) and her intracellular uric acid level indicated some stress on her body's ability to make antioxidants.

Although her total cholesterol level appeared slightly high, her good cholesterol (HDLs) is very good and this allowed the CRR (coronary risk ratio) to be ideal. Triglycerides are excellent at 0.5 indicating good carbohydrate selection and thus good quality HDL and LDL's. Statistically, it is highly unlikely she will ever have a heart problem if she continues with her current lifestyle. Low antioxidant production combined with vitamin D deficiency would make her more prone to cancer, statistically.

I seriously doubt if your doctor would interpret these laboratory results the way that I do, unless they are trained in anti-aging medicine, age management medicine, or health and longevity medicine.

"Remember, we are not only looking at the present "real time" state of health, we are also trying to predict any trends that may show problems in the future. Those problems can be contained, reversed, or eliminated when acted upon years or decades in advance.

HORMONE LABORATORY TESTS

HORMONES	F / M			1/4	2/4	3/4	4/4
T Testosterone	0.5-2.7 / 10-28	2.0f	16.0	1			
Free Testosterone	<50 / 250-800	700					
SHBG	20-90 / 9-60						
Free Androgen Index	<80 / >600	600					
PSA	0-4.0						
DHEA-S	2.0-12.0		5.2		1		
AoS/epiAos	<6.0		1.1				
P Cortisol	250-800	400	482			1	
IGF-1	80-400	>255	99	1			
IGF-BP3	2.1-4.8						
IGF-1/IGF-BP ratio	1.9-14.0						
Estradiol	90-1650 / 40-110	<50	704				
Progesterone	>15		60				

Estrogen/Progest ratio		20 120:1	11:1	1			
LH	2-100	>4.0	2.0				
FSH	2-115 / 40-110		2.3				
Free T 4	10-24.0	rx	12	1			
Free T 3	2.5-5.5	rx	4.2			1	
TSH	0.40-4.00		<0.06	1			

I determined by a hormonal assessment that this female patient was using testosterone cream inappropriately. Her well-meaning medical doctor had prescribed the cream without following up to see if the titrated dosage was correct. It was not. I fortunately caught this in time – this middle-aged female might have grown a mustache! There are additional side effects to high-level testosterone usage. The anabolic steroids used by some professional athletes are often 10 to 1000 times the normal dosage and can be deadly. It will devastate the hormonal system, liver, musculoskeletal system, etc.

The above list is not exhaustive. In a "general screening," it is an adequate assessment to see if appropriate levels are being achieved.

LABORATORY BLOOD SUGAR TESTS

BLOOD SUGAR	RANGE	IDEAL	RESULT	1/4	2/4	3/4	4/4
Glucose	3.5-6.0	<4.9	5.2			1	
HbA1C	4.4-6.4	<5, <30	5.2			1	
Insulin-P	10-80	<20	13				1
Triglycerides	<2.0		0.5				1

Fasting glucose is an indicator of many things. First, it tells us how much available sugar is circulating in the blood. Second, it informs us about how sensitive cell walls are to the effects of insulin, which removes glucose from the bloodstream. Lastly, it tells us about the free radical exposure created by normal and high levels of insulin and blood sugar, which can be fifty times more harmful than any other free radical made by the body. These are indicators of diabetes and pre-diabetes.

Another fact about blood glucose is that it tends to rise with age, like cholesterol. We know that when blood glucose rises above 5.1, one of the results of this higher-than-necessary level is the creation of free radicals called AGEs (accelerated glycosylated end products). In this process, glucose molecules attach to protein structures and cause the damage associated with biological aging. These AGEs put stress on the entire system, fueling silent inflammation and paving the road for obesity, "diabesity," and degenerative diseases.

Hemoglobin A1C is a wonderful test because it shows us *the average blood sugar level for the previous three months.* This is useful information because these levels are very important in their relationship to both serum insulin and glucose. If blood sugar is higher than hemoglobin A1C and insulin is low, it may point to pancreatic exhaustion. In other words, the pancreas is not producing enough insulin to keep blood sugar under control (there will usually be digestive complaints as well). If the reverse is true and the blood sugar level is lower than hemoglobin A1C, the patient may be prone to low blood sugar bouts of fatigue, mood changes, and sugar cravings.

The last possibility is most common and leads to metabolic syndrome; central obesity, heart disease (high cholesterol and oxidized LDLs), high blood sugar, high blood pressure, and possibly dementia. This is where insulin begins to skyrocket (called "insulin resistance") and the patient comes in saying, "I've tried every diet and nothing seems to work." This is very common as a precursor to diabetes – 30 percent of the US population has metabolic syndrome and an equal number in New Zealand and Australia.

High insulin levels are usually involved, and it works like this: The cells of the body that metabolize sugar to make energy become insensitive to insulin. These cells still require glucose to make energy, but it is stuck on the outside – insulin is the key to carrying sugar molecules from outside to inside the cell. So, if the cell is not listening ("resistant to insulin"), the pancreas turns up the volume by producing more insulin. Eventually, after five to 10 years of this process, pancreatic exhaustion and full-blown diabetes results. Patients who have enough sense to follow a low glycemic diet can usually correct this insulin insensitivity. The key is that it's a diet for life. Obesity associated with insulin resistance is often due to "leptin resistance." Without this fat-mobilizing hormone, you can gain weight on 500 calories per day. Now does it make sense why you cannot loose weight? Fix the insulin via diet, and you fix the leptin resistance.

Finally, my personal preference is to look at triglycerides in conjunction with the standard blood sugar tests. (And for you doctors, DHEA levels above the normal range is an indicator that the adrenal glands are in hyperplasia with correspondent metabolic stress. DHEA levels below the normal range will follow pancreatic exhaustion with high urate in most cases. This is why we checked all the tests.) Triglycerides are the only valid indicator of LDL and HDL particle size. Large "fluffy" LDL and HDL particles will stimulate the immune system, support repair, and cannot physically lodge in arteries to form plaque. Small, dense particles are oxidized and suppress immune function, and are associated with vascular pathology, mental decline, and a host of other maladies. Hydrogenated fats and high glucose are the primary offenders. *Robert Lustig, M.D. and pediatric endocrinologist, reports the fastest growing segment of the obese and oxidized population are six months to three years old! Ten-year-olds have arteriol damage or plaques commonly not seen until the fifties! I cannot state how important it is to control blood sugar to the range of 4.1 – 4.9 (< 86)*

GENERAL BLOOD COUNT AND SERUM CHEMISTRIES

BLOOD COUNTS	RANGE	IDEAL	RESULT	1/4	2/4	3/4	4/4
Red Cell Count	3.9-5.6		4.3				
Haemoglobin	115-155	137	130				
Haematocrit	0.35-0.45		0 . 3 9				1
Mean Cell Volume	80-100		92			1	
RDW	<15.0		13.9				
MPV	11.5-15 cent		10.3				
Platelets	150-450		232				
White Cell Count	4.0-11.0		5.1				
Neutrophils	2.0-8.0		3.2				
Lymphocytes	1.0-4.0		1.2		1		
Monocytes	0.0-1.0		0.36		1		
Eosinophils	0.0-0.5		0.36		1		
Basophils	0.0-0.2		0.05			1	
CHEMISTRIES							
Sodium	136-145		136				
Potassium	3.5-5.0		3.8				
Chloride	95-107		104				
Calcium	2.2-2.6		2.3/2.3				
Magnesium	0.6-1.2		0.8				
Creatinine	50-110		73				
Est GFR	80-120	85	79				
Urea	2.7-7.8		3.6			1	
Urate	0.14-0.37		0.25		1		
Bilirubin	3.0-21.0		8				
ALP	30-120		47				1
GGT	10.0-35		12				1
AST	10.0-50		18				1

ALT	0-40		18			1	
Albumin	35-50		44				
Protein	64-83		69				
Globulin			25				
A/G ratio	<2		1.76		1		
Vitamin D	50-150		46	1			
IMMUNOGLOBULINS							
IgA	0.8-3.5						
IgG	7.0-14.0	<8					
IgM	0.5-2.0						

You might suspect that "tired blood" and aging go along hand-in-hand? You would be correct; in men for instance, the red blood cell count tends to rise as we age. Because of high hemoglobin levels, excessive amounts of iron cause premature degeneration, liver damage, and ultimately death when people have confirmed "iron storage disease." What's alarming is that it's not that rare, and in my practice, I see men in their 50s and 60s pushing the top of the chart quite regularly. My best advice is to stay away from red meat (high source of iron) and give blood regularly – about four times per year. This little trick reduces a lot of free radical exposure to your body.

Your blood count is important for letting us understand how your red blood cells are maturing and that can be a great indicator of antioxidant load – or lack of it – and in general things like vitamin B12 and folic acid metabolism. Cholesterol composition and ratios within the blood are extremely important. Just as red blood cell counts tend to go up and bring more oxygen to cells that are getting older, white blood cells, platelets, and neutrophils tend to get lower.

This is dangerous because our immune system is made up of these components. Low white blood cell count and neutrophils predispose one to cancer, in addition to letting the histamine system go out of control, creating allergy and silent inflammation throughout the body. Simple things like hydration, good fiber intake, regular supplementation with high quality vitamins and minerals, in addition to a good night's sleep, will have a phenomenal effect on immune system competency. Normally we doctors look at this test for confirmation of infection, anemias, or other sinister processes. Using this test to make sure that the red cells are not too high and white cells are not too low is an important strategy.

When I'm fortunate enough to get to look at the laboratory work of somebody in their 80s and 90s, it's remarkable that they are so close to my ideals of a 25 to 35-year-old. They have slipped through the statistics because they are normal, but; they are statistically insignificant because they are not being tested as they are healthy and require 70-90 percent less health care throughout their life than the average population. *It seems ludicrous that we spend so much time studying disease without studying what actual healthy people do!* I know I'm not the first one to say this.

The serum chemistry is usually the last to change, meaning you have to be in fairly dire straits to push these tests far outside normal. The major electrolytes, sodium, potassium, chloride, calcium, and magnesium all are buffered within a very narrow range. The backup for these minerals is your bones. On a minute-by-minute basis, your bones are regulating your serum electrolytes. Without this fine regulation, your heart cannot function and your brain would quickly put you into seizures. Cramping and hyper agitation can be two signs of dehydration and are two very common symptoms that plague most people from time to time. Unless your symptoms are severe enough to get you into the emergency room, they will never be discovered. Drinking "hard water," and using real salt from the sea or deep mines all help with electrolyte balance.

Liver function tests, ALP, GGT, AST, ALT, on a subtle level, let us know about detoxification and overload of the liver. On a gross level, everything from hepatitis and parasites to alcoholism, the latter being quite common, can be picked up. ALT >25 can indicate fatty liver and under 40 is considered normal. Optimal levels are essential, as normal can kill you slowly as we have seen with blood sugar! Finally, the total protein levels are extremely important because they make up your immunoglobulins and these immune proteins are responsible for being the police to keep the bad guys at bay. We check every patient to make sure the protein ratios are in the correct range. Albumin to globulin ratio of 1.0 is ideal, greater than 2.0 shows stress and is of a concern to find out why the immune system is stressed.

Vitamin D may be one of the most important findings of the century. Author after author has sounded the bell of alarm to the scientific community.[6] Dr. Mercola, the internet health critic, stated, "The World

Health Organization recently attributed over 30 percent of the cancer deaths per year in the entire world to deficiencies in vitamin D."

With over 20 million deaths a year due to cancer and its terrible expressions, this leaves 6 million people possibly saved by the judicious use of lifestyle and one of the cheapest supplements available. Get your level tested, and stay in the upper quarter of the normal range. Get out in the sun 20 minutes a day!

---

[6] American Journal of Clinical Nutrition, Vol. 85, No. 6, 1586-1591, June 2007.

CHAPTER TWENTY-FOUR
Exercise – Motion Is Life

Just as the Heart, Cancer, and Diabetic associations provided overwhelming evidence that diet reduces your statistical probability of disease, they also support the same recommendations for exercise. Basically, they report, "Degenerative diseases are less in people who exercise regularly." "The Science" is definitive: this is a very effective drug!

How much exercise and what type is now much more specific to age, and can be tailored with respect to which diseases you may be more prone to. For instance, according to Dr. David Servan-Schreiber, M.D., "Studies show that physical exercise helps the body fight cancer. But the required dose is not the same for all cancers. Doses are calculated in MET units. For breast cancer, there seems to be a measurable effect after 3 to 5 hours per week of walking at a normal speed (equivalent to 9 METs per week). For cancer of the colon or rectum, twice as much (18 METs per week) is needed to have a comparable effect. This means either walking twice as long or twice as fast, or finding activities requiring more effort to replace walking. For example, bicycling at a speed that requires effort can add up to twice as many METs as walking.

How this doctor's recommendations translate to a "Stark Healthy Exercise" regime leaves little doubt that simplicity, discipline with regularity, and a passion for fun can all be a part of a disease-free "exercise lifestyle."

As the simplistic five, four, three, two, one approach to diet demonstrates, a minimum of one hour of exercise per day would lock in maximal benefit in disease prevention for most people. As some advanced disease-filled societies have obesity rates over 60 percent, I would recommend to anyone changing their exercise pattern to check-in with their healthcare professional and get the "All Clear" message before increasing activity. Post coronary bypass patients and patients who are in cancer therapy have all benefited from exercise. This is my personal experience and secondarily my professional experience with multiple patients. To be smart, be active!

The Facts About Exercise

As you grow older, the type of exercise you do has bearing on the body's response. It is generally accepted that a young and healthy 30-year-old can maintain optimal health and high performance values with about 70 percent of their activity on a weekly basis as aerobic. The other 30 percent should be confined to resistance training, flexibility and strength building exercises. When doing resistance training, be very focused on the amount of effort necessary to perform it. Resistance training is by far the most results-oriented of all exercises. You can build strength faster and change chemistry more quickly with 12 weeks of resistance training as opposed to any other method – especially as one ages.

As one grows older, we understand that the hormones in the aging body decline, making it more difficult to retain muscle mass. At the age of 50, we will have to devote 50 percent of our total workout time to resistance training to maintain a high level of performance. If you have maintained your fitness the previous two or three decades, the higher level of aerobic conditioning allows us to easily maintain cardiovascular efficiency and explosive power, and this yields a level of intensity in all that you do. The scale continues to slope towards resistance training as we age.

What a 70-year-old should be doing is about 70 percent resistance training. If we stick to our hour per day of exercise we can see a pattern. This pattern is easy to calculate for both men and women as to how much exercise and of what type is appropriate for their age group. Would you agree this is pretty simple?

Exercise does not just mean jogging and working out in the gym. I believe that being active outdoors is an exhilarating and engaging environment to maintain fitness. There's so much splendor to see in the environment.

Fitness itself is not a destination. It's a part of the culture where you live. It's part of your lifestyle that you share with friends and family. Exercise is as essential to a well-balanced life as a garden in the back-yard. Adaptability to the environment you live in is what is essential.

Well-earned vacations should be used as escapades of new and excit-ing activities that can expand upon your exercise baseline. While I myself spend time weekly in the gym and on the bike, I have another motive that drives me – to maintain my performance in the sports I have passion for such as paragliding, surfing, hiking and biking, yoga, martial arts, and whatever else looks like a lot of fun!

How privileged I am to have a good body that will allow me to do things that other people my age see as extreme or dangerous. I believe with the "Stark Healthy Exercise" guidelines you can main-tain a pain-free, high-performance body well into your 90s. In my sixties – so far I am as fit and flexible as a 30 year old. This is normal! We have the technology. The only question is do you have the desire to do it?

One of my colleagues in Age Management Medicine is Dr. Jeffry Life, M.D.; like myself, he found out the hard way that a life without exercise is a hard way of life! Take a look at his website and see what a 72-year-old can look like using the "Stark-Simple" guide-lines that I've given you. www.drlife.com

CHAPTER TWENTY-FIVE
Meditation – The "Brain Gym"

Starting from the mid 1960s, I have practised quite a few meditation techniques in my life. Some have been quite esoteric and others very simplistic and straightforward. To get the "physiological effect" on your brain and body, I have borrowed a method from the ancient masters. It gives a lifetime of benefit. To be fair, this meditative practice is only the beginning, or only an "induction" to deeper meditative practice.

I feel that if you're drawn to meditation you will look deeper and go further into more profound practices. There is no religious significance to what I'm teaching, and spiritual significance comes via confidence gained by personal experience. The brain itself demands attention and questions its own identity. Who actually is observing "self" and why is that significant? These are all questions that people should ask.

The platform of STARKHEALTH gives a solid base for people to take to their mere existence and project a meaning greater than the self. Meditation itself is a "mechanism," an internal exploration tool that can only be accomplished in a clear and uncluttered home. As with anything in the "StarkHealth Program," you will get out of it what you put into it. Approaching your meditation time with reverence and purpose will bring quick results.

Twice per day, 10 to 30 minutes is your time investment!

Meditation Practice

Regardless of the "brand" of meditation you use, the effects on the body, mind, and immune system are undeniable. When you meditate, make sure you follow these simple guidelines:

Rules Of Mindfulness

Meditation is a weight room workout for your mind. Meditation is not a nap and it is not a rest period (that is just a beneficial side effect). Let's go to the mind-gym!

PREPARATION

- Have a comfortable place to sit, in a warm room that is darkened or subdued. Stay away from draughts and open windows.

- Do some light stretches for your legs, lower back and shoulders. Let your body know it's time to be alert and mindful.

- Use a chair, cushion, pillow or block; whatever allows you to be undistracted, but remain upright in a comfortable seated position with legs crossed on the floor or in a chair.

- Settle into your seat, make sure your clothes are loose and do not constrict your body in any way. You may want to use a shawl or blanket around your shoulders.

- Take a few minutes and just sit. Let the mind calm down and the noise inside and outside be acknowledged and let go of completely. Loosen your muscles and joints until you are centered and comfortable.

- All meditation begins with the three following concepts:

- Right posture

- Right breathing

- Right thought

THE PRACTICE - "STARK OBSERVATION"

Whatever type of meditation you practise, begin here. If you only have five minutes, do it anyway. Twice a day for life, it's in the mind anyway.

If you do not have a meditation technique, try this ancient and dependable system: Observe the breath coming in the nose as you sit. Think to yourself, one breath in, one breath out, two breaths in, two breaths out, three breaths in, three breaths out...

When you get to ten, start over. Each round of ten is about one minute and 15 rounds of 10 are about right. (Thoughts will come and go so, if you are thinking about the parking meter, just say to yourself, "I am thinking about the parking meter. I will go back to my breathing now." Identify the distraction and return to breathing – it is very easy.) In addition, you can light an incense stick as they last about 30 to 40 minutes, so you have a timer that you can smell. Gently open your eyes, slowly do a couple of stretches and rejoin your day. The brain will reward you when you pay attention to its needs.

Meditation is the Royal Jelly of Consciousness!

CHAPTER TWENTY-SIX

Getting the Body Functioning: Pain Neutralization Therapy. The Kaufman Technique

Being a chiropractor and applied kinesiologist, I have a clear view of the body's structure and performance needs. In the beginning, as I mentioned before, my mentors were chiropractors and specialists in applied kinesiology. They taught me about the synergy of systems in the body, and how to go about integrating function.

The body trapped by pain and limitation of motion cannot have full organ or hormonal function by default. For the integration of my "Universal Theory of Aging" and the effects of declining hormones, we can generally say that people decline in movement and power as they age also. Most people would agree with this statement. On the other hand, I say this does not have to be true. You can have the strength, power, and movement of a young person at any age. I have proven this on myself and on my patients.

Pain Neutralization Therapy... "Wow! That's Amazing!"

Dr. Steven Kaufman, a Denver, Colorado, chiropractor, is another one of my colleagues. He's on the cutting edge of pain and mobility management with his newly defined "Pain Neutralization Technique." I have spent at least one week a year with Dr. Kaufman in Denver over the last five years to be brought up to speed in what

I consider the most revolutionary and effective physical medicine tool available. Removing pain within seconds and increasing mobility gently without "popping or clicking" can be done for a majority of patients quickly and efficiently.

Likewise, the method can be done for those with headaches, abdominal and vague pain syndromes and other problems. While not a panacea, it is in my view very revolutionary.

My advice is that if your body doesn't have the flexibility or movement of an active nubile 18-year-old, you need to see someone who can perform this advanced technique on you. You will then be able to function at a higher level internally and externally prepared for exercise and active engaged living. It's much like Mahatma Gandhi's saying, "Hungry people are not that interested in God – you have to feed them first." In as much, people who are in pain and have limited movement need to deal with that as a primary way back to health.

Check out my number one resource in this area to find a practitioner close to you who practises this gentle and effective technique: www. kaufmantechnique.com

CHAPTER TWENTY-SEVEN
Massage – A Touched Life!

My partner, Gayel, is one of the best massage therapists in the world. You might think that I'm a little biased, however, in my early days of practice, I spent a lot of time massaging my patients for their aches and pains. Massage itself is one of the oldest healing arts. Touch feels good. Children and animals that are not touched falter, while newborns have difficulty in life or do not survive at all. In our ever-expanding technology-based low-touch environments, massage becomes as essential as sunlight.

The physiological connection between a therapist and client is only one aspect of a massage therapy session. Another often-overlooked aspect of massage is the client has actually participated in making time in a busy day for themselves. This statement of self-worth is positive in the mental game of life.

Massage physically flushes the muscular system, greatly enhancing the movement of organic acids and lymphatic fluids. Thus, massage allows for quicker recovery from muscular activities such as exercise and a more complete and quicker response from the immune system when one is ill. (Can you think of any professional athletic team without a staff of massage therapists?) When you remove more toxins from the body and do it more quickly, you have a better chance of overcoming insults from bacteria, viruses, and environmental toxins with a medicine that actually feels good! It greatly helps to overcome all of these vectors of insult, ones that are uncountable in today's modern environment.

A weekly massage is not only recommended, I believe it's a necessity. No matter what style of massage you prefer, all will be beneficial to some degree. Find a therapist you like, one that leaves you feeling good and get started. Use your newfound exercise and dietary standards as a method to validate the reward of getting a massage once a week. Having something to look forward to is essential in health and longevity.

*As of late, I have been to see people in the hospital that are critically ill. When friends and relatives come in to the sterile environment, many walk right up to the patient with tubes and wires coming out of them and touch them, rub them and generally grab anything they can to connect. That is human and loving care at the same time. Sadly, the science does not see any use for it in hospital. Get it?

In my "life practice," it is massage first, chiropractic second, and drugs and surgery last!

CHAPTER TWENTY-EIGHT
The StarkHealth MATRIX from Complexity to Simplicity

Getting it all together does not have to be complex or overwhelming. Follow the matrix, which shows the essential, necessary points to receive your results.

Every part is simple and straightforward. Once you put them together, they become synergistic, magnifying, and empowering. The definition of synergy is a sum greater than the whole.

The irony here and my real lesson was that while I had the academic knowledge and my practice, "Synergy Health Center," in 1984, I did not put it into practice early enough to sidestep what could've been potentially deadly consequences. Balance is everything!

It's just 17 years until I will be 80. There is no guarantee that the hyper and fragmented early days of my life won't still come back to haunt me. However, everyday I do the very best I can to maintain optimal health as an investment in my longevity.

My goal is to be living to over 95 years, still physically active, mentally sharp, and independent. You're going to have to watch this space and see if my intentions and mechanisms will manifest. What's your goal, and how's your plan working for you?

As Rinpoche told me, I will tell you, "Please listen carefully to what I have said then apply it – go out and 'prove me wrong' with the work of your life; only then will you have experience and conviction to tell what you know."

INTENTIONS	+	MECHANISMS	=	RESULTS

S T A R K H E A L T H MATRIX
Complexity to Simplicity

Stark Reality Mindfulness	Stark Diet 5 Rules 4 Ever	Stark Movement Strength & Flow	Doctoring Monitoring

Age Management, Monitoring, Mentoring & Mastery   **StarkHealth**

	WHAT YOU DO 4 U		DOC's List	
K N O W L E D G E	Do 10-30 minutes of meditation twice per day. Two good times to do this are whilst waking and before the evening meal.	No junk foods 5 Veggies 4 Fruits 3 Proteins (palm size) 2 litres H2O 1 serving low GI grain Take Rx Vitamins	1 hr exercise/day 50% aerobic at 50, 40% at 60 years. Weight training, 3 to 4x/week Flexibility – Yoga/ Pilates 3x/week 1-2 longer outdoor adventures weekly	Measure Lab tests, Physical exam, Family history, Work environ, Stress assess	M E N T O R I N G
R E S U L T S	Increased concentration – focus and length of time. Better and faster recall	Reduced risk of disease, better energy and moods, younger-looking skin and better sexual function	Lower body fat, higher lean muscle mass, fewer injuries, faster healing, reduced blood sugar, better moods	Record rate of change, focus towards balance	M A S T E R Y

LIVE NOW – DIE LATER

PART FIVE

Epilogue. Last Thoughts for Today and Tomorrow

RESOURCES

Section A. Website Resources

Section B. References

Section C. Contact Details

EPILOGUE
Last Thoughts for Today and Tomorrow

As I continue to live each day with the excitement of being above ground, I give gratitude to those who make my day a joy and bless those who challenge me.

I vow to return with another book on how you as parents can protect your children's genes and decrease their rapid degeneration. I want to show you how to give them the life-saving skills they will need to survive in this most difficult of centuries.

All Blessings, ... I gotta FLY!

Patterson

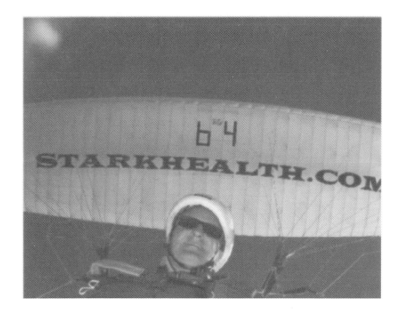

APPENDICES

Appendix A. Website Resources

Appendix B. References

Appendix C. Contact Information

APPENDIX A. WEBSITE RESOURCES

The Internet has made it easy for all of us to access information. Sometimes though, we wonder what that data actually means. Expertise is required when interpreting vast amounts of data, especially scientific data. Below you will find my recommendations for a concise focus on specific topics that make sense of the large amounts of data you need to master in this lifestyle renaissance called "STARKHEALTH."

LINKS

WWW.STARKHEALTH.COM

This is where it all began for me and discusses my quest to teach what I learned on my journey. On an island, at the top of the South Island of New Zealand, my website was born in 1996 You will find the mission statement of my life, plus interesting articles and resources for you and your families. I would recommend doing the "STARKHEALTH Analysis" as a place to begin. It is a very practical database of information specifically designed for you with recommendations on all the "Stark-things" that I have talked about in this book; it even gives you a specific nutraceutical prescription. This 10-to-20-page personal program is free to the world.

We try to make our programs accessible to as many people as possible. You can also purchase this book as a gift either in a digital version or as hardcopies. If you are going to the trouble to "pirate" a copy of the digital book, please don't. Just send me an email and tell me honestly why you cannot afford the low price and I will send you the digital book for free. It's not about the money, it's the message that I want to get out.

Finally, the website keeps you up-to-date with our work and how it is progressing. In the future, we plan to present "Lifestyle University," an interactive 2-3 day seminar where you actually learn all the fun things necessary to keep you and your family healthy by practicing them. Sound interesting? Watch this space. Sign up for our newsletter and get started on YOUR program. The clock is ticking!

WWW.LIVENOW-DIELATER.COM

Now you can get a digital copy of this book from our online store. You can also order copies of the paperback from associated retailers or direct from this website. We have many requests for multiple copies for companies and large families, so contact us via the website about our rates for volume and wholesale clients. This second edition will be available on Amazon in the USA and UK with their associated retailers. Keep up with the website from time to time as we may have some other languages available. Dr. Stark is also available worldwide on a limited basis for keynote addresses related to the Prevention, Performance, and Longevity paradigm.

WWW.IAPPL.CO.NZ (Want your healthcare provider to do this type of work?)

The International Academy of Prevention, Performance and Longevity: Prevention is the Cure, Lifestyle is our medicine!

This organization is the information highway for Dr. Stark's message. This is where the information is disseminated to the planet at large and it is done in three ways:

1. We train primary health care providers to use the tools of Lifestyle Medicine to clinically manage patients to Optimal Health and take control of their health risks and quality of life.

2. We train and care for Allied Health Care Professionals to engage, counsel and demonstrate how to achieve lasting pain free, disease free lives

3. We educate the public via our social media, outlets of information. Signup for our newsletters, online videos and become informed and involved in the future health of you and your loved ones.

WWW.KAUFMANTECHNIQUE.COM

Dr. Stephen Kaufman, D.C., is in my opinion the only true successor to Dr. George Goodheart. Goodheart created applied kinesiology in 1964 and passed away in 2008. He re-invented almost all of the paradigms we use in holistic care today. If you have ever seen a muscle test in a doctor's office, athletic setting, or at a health fair, Goodheart started it all. He was my first teacher, and between Doctors Goodheart, White, Walther, and Blaich, I amassed over 600 hours of personal instruction in the 1970s and 80s.

Dr. Kaufman is my contemporary and inspiration. Over the years we have been consistently involved with the development of our art and science. Dr. Kaufman has written over 70 professional papers and just in the last couple of years come into his own as a compassionate teacher. The concepts within "Pain Neutralization Therapy" are as revolutionary as Goodheart's concepts were 40 years ago.

Dr. Kaufman's website is a universe in itself. Please log on and have a look at what is coming in the next century. "We really can stop pain in 30 seconds ... not in all, but in a majority of our patients."
–Kaufman

WWW.WORLDHEALTH.NET

The American Academy of Anti-Aging Medicine. As a certified diplomate of the American Board of Anti-Aging Health Practitioners, I feel they are at the forefront of the professional advancement in this field. Over the last 18 years, they have gone from a dozen physicians to over 18,000 members worldwide! Their world congresses held twice a year are the place to be for cutting-edge research on human aging and performance. The site itself is an excellent reference for any and all interested in enhancing their quality of daily life: anti-aging lifestyles.

WWW.NUTRIWEST.COM

Nutri-West, Douglas, Wyoming. This is one of the first nutrition companies to set the professional standards we look for today. They have worked with the FDA to help create the Goods and Manufacturing Practices code, which sets the highest standard for the making of the nutraceuticals we use. The Clinical Nutrition formulations are from consulting physicians in the field and have been proven to work over time. I have contributed formulations to aid my fellow doctors and patients over the years. This is also the company whose products I personally used when overcoming terminal cancer. Yes, I know Dr. Paul and Marcia White and their lovely family personally; it is refreshing to know a handshake with that family on any issue is as good as any corporate seal and always will be.

DISCLAIMER: Financial interest. In order to have access to the best products in the world from my location in New Zealand, at the request of the Whites', I personally became the distributor of these products for New Zealand and Australian health practitioners. I use multiple companies' products for my private practice; however, these are among the best I have ever found and make up the core of the products I use.

WWW.DRSIMONE.COM

Charles B. Simone, M.MS., M.D. It is rare to come into contact with a champion and see that the person is a champion immediately. I met Dr. Simone at the American Academy of Anti-Aging Medicine after a breathtaking lecture to 5,000 doctors. As a researcher and clinician in the cancer and immunology field, he is at the forefront of the war on cancer. His compassion and common sense have made remarkable contributions to the lives of many, many patients. He is an authority as an oncologist and nutritionist, showing the profession how antioxidant therapy in conjunction with chemotherapy helps and does not hinder outcomes. His site is humble as he is; you would not expect the benefits that you get by learning from Dr. Simone.

WWW.MENDOSA.COM

David Mendosa is a master of information technology. His passion is the glycemic index and glycemic load, and the effects of carbohydrate foods on insulin, diabetes, and quality of life. As most of anti-aging medicine is concerned first and foremost with insulin levels, this link is a must-go-to when you want to learn about the topic.

WWW.VIRTUALMEDITATION.COM

Stephen Sinatra (Dr. Sinatra's son) is one of our favorite people. He is a dedicated "Foodie" and ingenious nutritionist and devoted meditator. His website is a fantastic resource for easy to follow meditative instruction and motivation. To know Stephen is to love life.

WWW.DRSINATRA.COM

Dr. Sinatra is my personal friend and mentor. This website is "a cardiologist's Guide to Total Wellness." Dr. Sinatra has been educating via newsletters to the public, and lecturing to his peers for over 15 years. He is the author of countless health articles, and several excellent books, a ready and regular reference in your personal library. I really recommend his newsletter, as it is a must for anyone with heart disease under standard treatment. Get involved and be informed and you will benefit.

WWW. GROUNDED.COM

Another wonderful concept pioneered by doctor Sinatra. It is a scientifically proven method of resetting the electromagnetics of the body and reducing killer chronic inflammation. Get informed and get outside!

WWW.FREEFALLEXPERIENCE.COM

If you are interested in actualizing your dreams and experiencing a different way of being, the Freefall Experience® is for you! I have been to Sally's workshops; she gets to the bottom of why people do not demand action in their life. She's a personal coach for the Chairman of the Board or those needing a high level of target-specific action. Sally is the real deal.

As she says; "Most people rely on external circumstances shifting in order to gauge how HAPPY they are."

This isn't it yet; there's somewhere else to get! When I get "there," it will be better.... But where is this place called "THERE"?

During the Freefall Experience®, you will examine the beliefs and behaviors that have hindered you from achieving what you want in your life. This unique education is not for the faint-hearted. It is designed for those who are truly interested in leading an extraordinary existence.

WWW.WESTONAPRICE.ORG

This is the modern home of the work which began my lifelong work and program back to health. Read Sally Fallon's books, give them to your children when they move from home or go to college. This is the fundamental work you need to know. I cannot overstate how important it is.

WWW.BUY1-GIVE1FREE.COM

The Power of WOW, WOOOW! Every time you buy one of these books, a child gets access to clean water. We are proud members of "B1G1," and now you are too via your association with "StarkHealth". Make your act of giving related to each transaction and see how quickly a few can affect the many. Check it out, it will change lives today!

APPENDIX B. REFERENCES

1. JAMA, July 7, 1989.

2. Kuler, L, et al. Circulation 1966; 34:1056

3. Too much revascularization? Scientific American Vol. 17: March/ April 1994.

4. 4. Herrick JB, JAMA, 1912; 59: 2015.

5. White, PD My Life in Medicine: An Autobiographical Memoir. Boston, MA: Gambit & Co. 1971.

6. Price WA, Nutrition and Physical Degeneration. New Canaan, Ct: Keats Publishing, Inc. 1989.

7. Rothernburg, R, et al. Forever Ageless: Advanced edition. Encinitas, Ca.: Published by California Health Span Institute.

8. Segal S, et al. Male hyperprolactimenic effects on infertility. Fertility and Sterility, 1979; 32:556-559.

9. Alexander GM, et al. Testosterone and sexual behaviour in oral contraceptive users and non-users. Horm Behav, 1990; 24:388-402.

10. Kirby RS et al (eds). Impotence, Oxford: Butterworth-Heinemann, 1991.

11. Seaman B. The Doctors' Case Against The Pill, PH Wyden, 1969.

12. Matsumoto AM, Brenner WJ. Parallel dose-dependant suppression of LH, FSH and sperm production by testosterone in normal men. Abstract No. 570, Proceeding of the 70th Annual Meeting of the Endocrine Society, 1988; The Endocrine Society, Bethesda, MD.

13. World Heath Organization www.who.int/mediacentre/ news/releases/2003/pr27/ en/

14. Pikarsky E et al. NF-kappaB functions as a tumour promoter in inflammation-associated cancer. Nature. 2004 Sep 23; 431(7007): 46 1-6. Epub Aug 25, 2004.

APPENDIX C. CONTACT INFORMATION

We are very lucky to attract a wonderful group of clients from around the world. Our busy research practice still enjoys seeing new patients who want to capture the essence of Prevention, Performance, and Longevity in their life. Over the phone, or Skype, we talk about life, get traction on issues, and push the "happy" envelope every day.

I expect to do this for another 50 years, so if you are really moved to see me personally, give me a call. We may find room for you. We hold the practice as a teaching forum and limit client numbers to 50 per year, not the 2,000 to 3,000 of a normal doctors' practice. Slow food – slow doctors! The good news is we are training other providers to do the Stark Health Program for you in your area! Just ask us who we have trained and hopefully they will be in your area. Become a member of the IAPPL and stay informed and in action more importantly.

For more information or to book speaking engagements that motivate your audience to take action and improve their health today, email me at starkhealthcentre@mac.com

You may always reach me through my website:
WWW.STARKHEALTH.COM

- Do our health and lifestyle analysis online,

- Send this book to your friends and loved ones (you can by it online at our website)

- Join the IAPPL (International Academy of Prevention, Performance and Longevity) Lifestyle Medicines pipeline for the latest information and inspiration: www.IAPPL.co.nz

- Get involved with your outcome!

- Live Now – Die Later, on your terms!

I want to hear from you. Were you inspired after reading my book? Let me know. Do you need a little encouragement on your health pathway? Send me an email. I'll connect with you and give you further resources that will help.

Start Here with the "Stark Truths" about Your Health.

	PHYSICAL	CHEMICAL	MENTAL
Base line Measure-ments, where you are at NOW Test, Measure and Record	Ht Wt BMI Waist Hips Legs Arms VO2Max Body Fat% Body H2O%	Cholesterol, LDL, HDL TRIGS CRP-hsCBC Cortisol Testosterone Estrogen Vitamin D Growth Hormone **SYSTEMS NEEDING SUPPORT**	Moods Concentration Clarity of thought Interactiveness Quality sleep hours? Laughing daily? Stress levels Quality of Life
90 DAYS Tools, diet, exercise, Nutriceuticals, Lab tests	Body Remeasure and record every 90 days	Retest specific labs **CORRECTION**	Reassess and Record
LONG TERM Retest and record every 90 days	Remeasure and record every 90 days	Retest your labs yearly **PERFECTION**	Reassess and Record

Test, Measure and Record your Physical Statistics, Blood Chemistry, and Mental State in the sections provided. You may need the help of a Personal Trainer, Nurse, or Medical Practitioner.

Adopt the recommended actions from the Stark Health Matrix on page 269.

Live long and well. It's a choice.